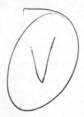
Independent Inquiry into
Inequalities in Health
REPORT

LONDON: TSO

Published by TSO (The Stationery Office) and available from:

Online
www.tso.co.uk/bookshop

Mail, Telephone, Fax & E-mail
TSO
PO Box 29, Norwich NR3 1GN
Telephone orders/General enquiries 0870 600 5522
Fax orders 0870 600 5533
Email book.orders@tso.co.uk
Textphone 0870 240 3701

TSO Shops
123 Kingsway, London WC2B 6PQ
020 7242 6393 Fax 020 7242 6394
68-69 Bull Street, Birmingham B4 6AD
0121 236 9696 Fax 0121 236 9699
9-21 Princess Street, Manchester M60 8AS
0161 834 7201 Fax 0161 833 0634
16 Arthur Street, Belfast BT1 4GD
028 9023 8451 Fax 028 9023 5401
18-19 High Street, Cardiff CF10 1PT
029 2039 5548 Fax 029 2038 4347
71 Lothian Road, Edinburgh EH3 9AZ
0870 606 5566 Fax 0870 606 5588

TSO Accredited Agents
(See Yellow Pages)

and through good booksellers

First published 1998
Sixth impression 2005

ISBN 0 11 322173 8

Printed in the United Kingdom by The Stationery Office
180341 C3 7/05 311011

INDEPENDENT INQUIRY INTO INEQUALITIES IN HEALTH

The Inquiry was chaired by:

Sir Donald Acheson, Chairman of the International Centre for Health and Society at University College, London.

Scientific Advisory Group

The Inquiry was overseen by a Scientific Advisory Group.

The members of the Group were:

Professor David Barker FRS,
Director of the Medical Research Council's Environmental Epidemiology Unit,
University of Southampton

Dr Jacky Chambers,
Director of Public Health, Birmingham Health Authority

Professor Hilary Graham,
Director of the Economic and Social Research Council's Health Variations Programme,
Lancaster University

Professor Michael Marmot,
Director of the International Centre for Health and Society, University College, London

Dr Margaret Whitehead,
Visiting Fellow, the King's Fund, London

Secretariat

Administrative Secretary:
Dr Ray Earwicker, seconded from the Department of Health

Scientific Secretary:
Dr Catherine Law, seconded from the Medical Research Council's Environmental Epidemiology Unit, University of Southampton

Statistical Adviser:
Frances Drever, seconded from the Office for National Statistics

THE INQUIRY'S TERMS OF REFERENCE

1. To moderate a Department of Health review of the latest available information on inequalities of health, using data from the Office for National Statistics, the Department of Health and elsewhere. The data review would summarise the evidence of inequalities of health and expectation of life in England and identify trends.

2. In the light of that evidence, to conduct – within the broad framework of the Government's overall financial strategy – an independent review to identify priority areas for future policy development, which scientific and expert evidence indicates are likely to offer opportunities for Government to develop beneficial, cost effective and affordable interventions to reduce health inequalities.

3. The review will report to the Secretary of State for Health. The report will be published and its conclusions, based on evidence, will contribute to the development of a new strategy for health.

Preface

This Report addresses an issue which is fundamentally a matter of social justice; namely that although the last 20 years have brought a marked increase in prosperity and substantial reductions in mortality to the people of this country as a whole, the gap in health between those at the top and bottom of the social scale has widened. Yet there is convincing evidence that, provided an appropriate agenda of policies can be defined and given priority, many of these inequalities are remediable. The same is true for those that exist between the various ethnic groups and between the sexes.

In July 1997, I was invited by the Secretary of State for Health to review and summarise inequalities in health in England and to identify priority areas for the development of policies to reduce them. To accomplish this task, I have been aided by a small group of scientists. This Report is the result of our work together.

In this work, we have consulted widely and drawn on the expertise of a range of colleagues whose names are acknowledged in the Report. We also acknowledge and have built on the work of those who have gone before us. We mention in particular Sir Douglas Black's ground breaking report "Inequalities in Health". We have also found inspiration in the work of the World Health Organisation which, in its European "Health for All" Policy, gives precedence above all other objectives to the promotion of equity in health within and between countries.

There have been many relevant developments between the appointment of the Inquiry and our submission of this Report to Ministers. From its earliest days in office, the Government has expressed its concern about inequalities in health and in February 1998 translated this concern into a central premiss of its consultation paper "Our Healthier Nation". This has been followed not only by the 1998 Budget but by a succession of consultation documents and White Papers relevant to our inquiry.

As our work developed, it has become clear that the range of factors influencing inequalities in health extends far beyond the remit of the Department of Health and that a response by the Government as a whole will be needed to deal with them.

We believe that the policies and areas for policy development which we have identified from the available evidence, comprise an effective agenda. Its components are congruent and mutually reinforcing. We are convinced that if this agenda is implemented it will make a major beneficial impact on inequalities in health. We hope that it will also provide a sound basis for policy development well into the next millennium.

At this point, the scientific work of the Inquiry is done. We commend the Report to the elected Government as a significant contribution to social equity worthy of urgent consideration. It is now for the Government to decide the rate of implementation and the affordability of our recommendations.

Sir Donald Acheson

September 1998

Contents

List of Tables and Figures

TABLES

FIGURES

Synopsis

Our task has been to review the evidence on inequalities in health in England, including time trends, and, as a contribution to the development of the Government's strategy for health, to identify areas for policy development likely to reduce these inequalities. We carried out our task over the last 12 months, drawing on scientific and expert evidence, and peer review.

Although average mortality has fallen over the past 50 years, unacceptable inequalities in health persist. For many measures of health, inequalities have either remained the same or have widened in recent decades.

These inequalities affect the whole of society and they can be identified at all stages of the life course from pregnancy to old age.

The weight of scientific evidence supports a socioeconomic explanation of health inequalities. This traces the roots of ill health to such determinants as income, education and employment as well as to the material environment and lifestyle. It follows that our recommendations have implications across a broad front and reach far beyond the remit of the Department of Health. Some relate to the whole Government while others relate to particular Departments.

We have identified a range of areas for future policy development, judged on the scale of their potential impact on health inequalities, and the weight of evidence. These areas include: poverty, income, tax and benefits; education; employment; housing and environment; mobility, transport and pollution; and nutrition. Areas are also identified by the stages of the life course – mothers, children and families; young people and adults of working age; and older people – and by focusing on ethnic and gender inequalities. We identify possible steps within the National Health Service to reduce inequalities. In our view, these areas offer opportunities over time to improve the health of the less well off.

There are three areas which we regard as crucial:
• all policies likely to have an impact on health should be
    evaluated in terms of their impact on health inequalities;
• a high priority should be given to the health of families with children;
• further steps should be taken to reduce income inequalities and improve the living
    standards of poor households.

These areas form the basis of our first three recommendations.

We hope our report will provide a sound basis for policy development well into the next millennium.

Donald Acheson

David Barker

Jacky Chambers

Hilary Graham

Michael Marmot

Margaret Whitehead

PART 1

Introduction

Our Task

Our task is set out in the terms of reference and the commissioning letter from the Minister for Public Health (annex A). It consists of two parts. The first is to review the latest available information on health inequalities and "*summarise the evidence of inequalities of health and the expectation of life in England and identify trends*". This review would be based on data from the Office for National Statistics (ONS), the Department of Health (DH) and elsewhere.

The second is to identify, in the light of the review, "*priority areas for future policy development . . . likely to offer opportunities for Government to develop beneficial, cost effective and affordable interventions to reduce health inequalities*". These policy proposals are to be based on "*scientific and expert evidence*" and "*within the broad framework of the Government's financial strategy*".

Bearing in mind the commissioning letter and terms of reference, we have considered the work of the Inquiry to be scientific. We have limited our recommendations to those based on scientific and expert evidence.

The short timescale of the Inquiry, combined with the broad nature of inequalities in health and their determinants, prohibited a very detailed and comprehensive review. We acknowledge at the outset of this report that there are areas which, given a longer period of time for our work, we would have reviewed in more detail. Other areas of work were omitted because they were not included in our terms of reference. So, although we recognise that the setting of targets concerned with reducing inequalities in health is an important area for policy development, we were advised that consideration of this issue was not within the Inquiry's remit. We do, however, welcome the setting up of the Chief Medical Officer's working group which will consider targets, including those which address inequalities in health, as part of the work on "Our Healthier Nation"[1]. In addition, we decided at an early stage not to consider recommendations for research and development, although the need for further research and development is implicit in many sections of the report.

A key objective of our report is to contribute to the development of the Government's strategy for health and an agenda for action on inequalities in the longer term. The publication on the 5 February 1998 of the consultation paper "Our Healthier Nation; a Contract for Health"[1] was an important landmark. It identified the need "*to improve the health of the worst off in society and to narrow the health gap*" as an overriding principle. This principle also underpins consultation papers on public health from Scotland, Wales and Northern Ireland[2-4].

Our report takes account of the main features of "Our Healthier Nation" as they affect inequalities. We discuss tackling inequalities in the settings of schools, the workplace and neighbourhoods. Our section on the NHS includes an element on the reduction of inequalities through local partnerships taking account of plans for Health Improvement Programmes and Health Action Zones. It also takes into account the changes outlined in the White Paper "*The New NHS: Modern and Dependable*"[5].

Structure of the report

Our report is divided into two sections. Part 1 sets out the approach which we adopted in considering the causes of inequalities in health, and some of the principles which have guided our work. This is followed by a summary of our review of data on inequalities in health, "The Current Position". Part 2 is our review of the evidence from which we identified areas for future policy development, and contains our recommendations. This section also adds to, and amplifies, some of the data presented in Part 1. In each of the identified areas for future policy development, we have summarised the inequalities that exist, the evidence that indicates areas for policy development, and the benefit which might result from such development. A complete list of our recommendations, including cross references, is given at the end of Part 2.

Our approach

Historical context

Our report needs to be seen in its historical context, as an extension of scientific and policy development in this country over more than a century. There is a long tradition in Britain of analysing national statistics to shed light on the nature and causes of social inequalities in health[6]. This goes back at least to William Farr in 1837, when the General Register Office was set up. Farr, as the first Superintendent of Statistics, clearly believed that it was the responsibility of the national office not just to record deaths, but to uncover underlying linkages which might help to prevent disease and suffering in the future[7].

Firm foundations were set at that time which have allowed the documentation and monitoring of health inequalities over the past 150 years to a much finer degree than in many other countries. Social and public health reformers since then – from Chadwick in the 1840s to Rowntree at the turn of the century and Titmuss and colleagues in the Depression and post-war period – have carried on the tradition, bringing the evidence into the light of day for public debate and action.

Evidence on social inequalities and of inadequate access to health care in Britain also played a key role in pressure to set up the welfare state in the post-war period, with the landmark Beveridge Report of 1942 setting out a national programme of policies and services to combat the "five giants of Want, Disease, Ignorance, Squalor and Idleness"[8].

It was an assessment in the mid-1970s that Britain was slipping behind some other countries in health improvement, despite 30 years of the welfare state, and speculation that persisting health inequalities were to blame, that led to the setting up by the Government of the Research Working Group on Inequalities in Health in 1977, chaired by Sir Douglas Black. The resulting Black Report[9] presented in 1980, shortly after a new Government took office, was a rare example, perhaps the first anywhere in the world, of an attempt authorised by Government to explain trends in inequalities in health and relate these to policies intended to promote as well as restore health[10]. The thrust of the recommendations in that seminal report were concerned with improving the material conditions of life of poorer groups, especially children and people with disabilities, coupled with a re-orientation of health and personal social services. Although there was little sign that the report's recommendations were given any official priority in Britain throughout the 1980s, ripples from the report spread out far and wide, to be influential in research and public health debates in many countries. For example, the Black Report played a part in influencing the decision of the member states (including the UK) of the European Region of the World Health Organisation to agree a common health strategy in 1985, with equity in health as a theme running right through it, and reduction in inequities as the subject of the first of 38 targets to be achieved by the year 2000[11]. This in itself has proved a significant development on the international front. In 1987, an update of the evidence in the Black Report was commissioned and published under the title of "The Health Divide"[12]. This stimulated widespread debate and led to renewed calls for greater priority to be given to the issue of inequalities in health[10].

It was not until the 1990s, however, that significant movement on the issue was perceptible. The Chief Medical Officer for England set up a sub-group under the auspices of "The Health of the Nation" national health strategy, to look into what the Department of Health and the NHS could do to reduce variations in health[13]. The report of the sub-group was published in 1995, and in the same year, the King's Fund published an independent analysis of the wider policy options for tackling inequalities in health in relation to housing, family poverty, and smoking as well as the NHS[14]. These initiatives, together with a growing body of evidence from a great many in the public health field, were influential in convincing the new Government in 1997 of the need to set up the current Independent Inquiry.

Socioeconomic model of health

We have adopted a socioeconomic model of health and its inequalities. This is in line with the weight of scientific evidence. Figure 1 shows the main determinants of health as layers of influence, one over another[15,16]. At the centre are individuals, endowed with age, sex and constitutional factors which undoubtedly influence their health potential, but which are fixed. Surrounding the individuals are layers of influence that, in theory, could be modified. The innermost layer represents the personal behaviour and way of life adopted by individuals, containing factors such as smoking habits and physical activity, with the potential to promote or damage health. But individuals do not exist in a vacuum: they interact with friends, relatives and their immediate

Figure 1: The main determinants of health. Concentric arcs labelled from outermost to innermost: General socioeconomic, cultural and environmental conditions; Living and working conditions (Work environment, Unemployment, Education, Water & Sanitation, Health care services, Agriculture and food production, Housing); Social and community networks; Individual lifestyle factors; Age, sex and constitutional factors.

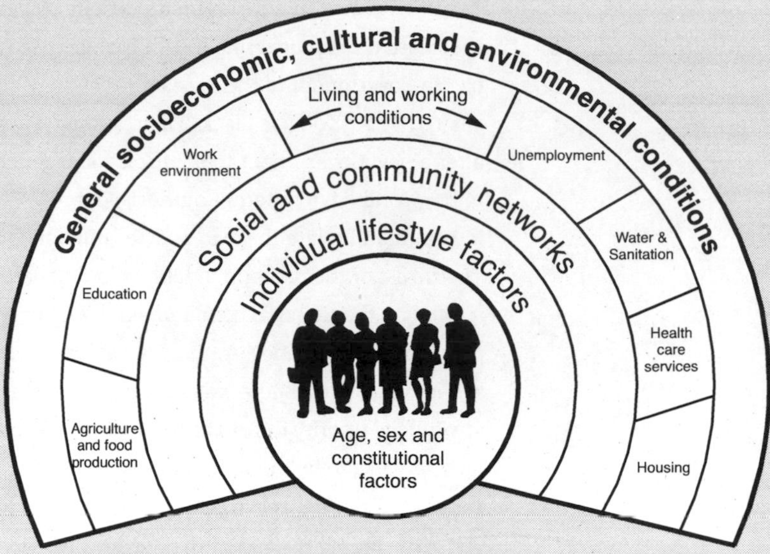

community, and come under the social and community influences represented in the next layer. Mutual support within a community can sustain the health of its members in otherwise unfavourable conditions. The wider influences on a person's ability to maintain health (shown in the third layer) include their living and working conditions, food supplies and access to essential goods and services. Overall there are the economic, cultural and environmental conditions prevalent in society as a whole, represented in the outermost layer.

The model emphasises interactions between these different layers. For example, individual lifestyles are embedded in social and community networks and in living and working conditions, which in turn are related to the wider cultural and socioeconomic environment.

Socioeconomic inequalities in health reflect differential exposure – from before birth and across the life span – to risks associated with socioeconomic position. These differential exposures are also important in explaining health inequalities which exist by ethnicity and gender. One model of how these risks interconnect is shown in figure 2.

This model has been used to guide research. The research task is to trace the paths from social structure, represented by socioeconomic status, through to inequalities in health. This can be done in stages, for example showing that work is related to pathophysiological changes such as raised blood pressure or biochemical disturbances which are in turn related to disease risk; or showing that the social environment in which people live is related to their health behaviour, such as patterns of eating, drinking, smoking and physical activity.

The model also illustrates various intervention points. Medical care, for example, might intervene at the level of morbidity to prevent progression to death, or earlier, at the level of pathophysiological changes to interrupt transition to morbidity.

Figure 2

**Socioeconomic circumstances
and health outcomes**

Source:
International Centre for Health and Society,
University College, London, unpublished (1998)

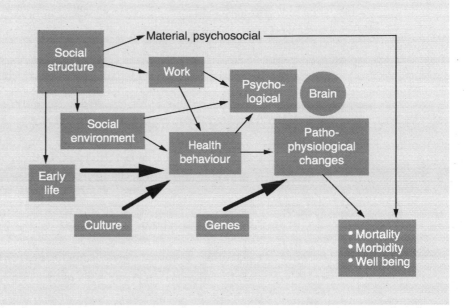

Preventive approaches might act at the level of attempting to change individual risk, by encouraging people to give up smoking or change diet. Interventions in the workplace or the social environment might encourage a climate which promotes healthy behaviour or improved psychological conditions. Interventions at the level of social structure would reduce social and economic inequalities.

Our approach is shared by the Government which, in "Our Healthier Nation", has expressed its determination to tackle "*the root causes of health*". The Prime Minister emphasised this approach in his answer to a Parliamentary Question on low income, inequality and health (11th June 1997).

> ". . . It is for that reason that the Secretary of State for Health has asked Sir Donald Acheson to conduct a further review into inequality and the link between health and wealth ....
> These inequalities do matter and there is no doubt that the published statistics show a link between income, inequality and poor health. It is important to address that issue, and we are doing so. The purpose of the windfall tax is to address that matter on behalf of young people and the long-term unemployed. We are also addressing the issue by introducing the minimum wage, which will help those on low incomes, and with welfare measures, particularly those designed to get single parents back to work"[17].

Need to intervene on a broad front

The socioeconomic model also dictates the breadth of our review. A broad front approach reflects scientific evidence that health inequalities are the outcome of causal chains which run back into and from the basic structure of society. Such an approach is also necessary because many of the factors are interrelated. It is likely to be less effective to focus solely on one point if complementary action is not in place which influences a linked factor in another policy area. Policies need to be both "upstream" and "downstream".

For instance, a policy which reduces inequalities in income and improves the income of the less well off, and one which provides pre-school education for all four year olds are examples of "upstream" policies which are likely to have a wide range of consequences, including benefits to health. Policies such as providing nicotine replacement therapy on prescription, or making available better facilities for taking physical exercise, are "downstream" interventions which have a narrower range of benefits.

We have, therefore, recommended both "upstream" and "downstream" policies – those which deal with wider influences on health inequalities such as income distribution, education, public safety, housing, work environment, employment, social networks, transport and pollution, as well as those which have narrower impacts, such as on healthy behaviours. We describe the impact of these on health at the various stages of the life course, by ethnicity and by gender.

Absolute and relative inequalities

The health gap between socioeconomic groups can be considered in both relative and absolute terms. An example of a relative measure would be the ratio of the death rate in the lowest social class to that in the highest class. Death rates could be, for example, twice as high in the lowest as in the highest social class. The equivalent absolute measure would subtract the death rate in one group from that in another to give the rate difference. This could be expressed as, for example, the death rate in the lowest social class is 50 deaths per 100,000 population greater than the rate in the highest social class.

Both relative and absolute measures have important implications. However, it may be argued that absolute measures are the most critical, particularly with respect to identifying the major problems which need to be addressed. This is because an absolute measure is determined not only by how much more common the health problem is in one group than another, but also how common the underlying problem – for example the death rate in a particular population – actually is. A doubling in social class V of the rate of occurrence of a rare disease is not as significant as a doubling in the rate of occurrence of a common disease. Major gains in attacking health inequalities are most likely to derive from addressing those health problems which occur reasonably frequently, even if less common diseases may in relative terms demonstrate a steep gradient, occurring, say, ten or twenty times more often in social class V than I. Relative measures are particularly useful for assessing the relative importance of different causal factors, and are important tools in aetiological enquiry.

The penalties of inequalities in health affect the whole social hierarchy and usually increase from the top to the bottom. Thus, although the least well off may properly be given priority, if policies only address those at the bottom of the social hierarchy, inequalities will still exist. Accordingly, our approach addresses the socioeconomic determinants of health as they affect the whole social spectrum.

Social environment, social support and health

The economic and social benefits of greater equality seem to go hand in hand. The quality of the social environment is worst where financial deprivation is greatest, such as the inner cities. Recent research suggests that, in addition to the ill effects due to absolute poverty, societies in which there is a wide gap between the rich and the poor suffer additional social problems, for instance, through high rates of violence and crime, and truancy[18]. It has also been suggested that people with good social networks live longer, are at reduced risk of coronary heart disease, are less likely to report being depressed, or to suffer a recurrence of cancer and are less susceptible to infectious illness than those with poor networks[19].

This work opens up a range of policy options. Policies to reduce social inequalities and to promote social networks are part of a strategy to reduce inequalities in health in just the same way as action on economic inequalities or improvements in the material environment of disadvantaged communities. These include, for instance, policies which reduce unemployment in areas of social need, those which improve the availability of social housing for families close to their social networks, and the provision of family support services which help parents protect their children from the effects of disadvantage. Freedom from prejudice or discrimination, a respect for individual worth and a sense of belonging to society will help to reduce the manifestations of exclusion, such as crime, violence, self-harm and isolation.

Priority for parents and children

While remediable risk factors affecting health occur throughout the life course, childhood is a critical and vulnerable stage where poor socioeconomic circumstances have lasting effects. Follow up through life of successive samples of births has pointed to the crucial influence of early life on subsequent mental and physical health and development[20]. The fact that the adverse outcomes, for example, mental illness, short stature, obesity, delinquency and unemployment, cover a wide range, carries an important message. It suggests that policies which reduce such early adverse influences may result in multiple benefits, not only throughout the life course of that child but to the next generation.

Another line of research, which concentrates on the effects of a mother's nutrition on her child's later health, has shown that small size or thinness at birth are associated with coronary heart disease, diabetes and hypertension in later life. As two principal determinants of a baby's weight at birth are the mother's pre-pregnant weight and her own birthweight, the need for policies to improve the health of (future) mothers and their children is obvious[21]. It also follows that, among migrants who move from a poorly nourished to a well nourished community, there will be implications for fetal growth and adult health for more than one generation.

Taking into account these findings and the view expressed in "Our Healthier Nation" that "*good health is the supreme gift parents can give their children*", we take the view that, while there are many potentially beneficial interventions to reduce inequalities in health in adults of working age and older people, many of those with the best chance of reducing future inequalities in mental and physical health relate to parents, particularly present and future mothers, and children.

Inequalities in Health: The Current Position

Intro

Socioeconomic inequalities in health and expectation of life have been found in many contemporary and past societies. In England although information based on an occupational definition of social class has only been available since 1921, other data identifying differences in longevity by position in society have been available for at least two hundred years. These differences have persisted despite the dramatic fall in mortality rates over the last century[6].

Inequalities in health exist, whether measured in terms of mortality, life expectancy or health status; whether categorised by socioeconomic measures or by ethnic group or gender. Recent efforts to compare the level and nature of health inequalities in international terms indicate that Britain is generally around the middle of comparable western countries, depending on the socioeconomic and inequality indicators used[22]. Although in general disadvantage is associated with worse health, the patterns of inequalities vary by place, gender, age, year of birth and other factors, and differ according to which measure of health is used[23].

General trends in health

Death rates in England have been falling over the last century, from a crude death rate of 18 per thousand people in 1896 to 11 per thousand in 1996[24,25]. Over the last 25 years, there have been falls in death rates from a number of important causes of death, for example lung cancer (for men only), coronary heart disease and stroke[25].

Life expectancy has risen over the last century[26], but not all life is lived in good health. Healthy life expectancy – the measure of average length of life free from ill health and disability – has not been rising; the added years of life have been years with a chronic illness or disability[27].

The proportion of people reporting a limiting long standing illness has risen from 15 per cent to 22 per cent since 1975. The proportion reporting illness in the two weeks previous to interview has nearly doubled from 9 per cent to 16 per cent. There is a slight increase in the proportion of people consulting the NHS[28].

Measuring socioeconomic position

A number of different measures can be used to indicate socioeconomic position. These include occupation, amount and type of education, access to or ownership of

	Social Class		Occupation
I	**Professional**		accountants, engineers, doctors
II	**Managerial & Technical/**		marketing & sales managers, teachers,
	Intermediate		journalists, nurses
IIIN	**Non-manual Skilled**		clerks, shop assistants, cashiers
IIIM	**Manual Skilled**		carpenters, goods van drivers, joiners, cooks
IV	**Partly Skilled**		security guards, machine tool operators, farm workers
V	**Unskilled**		building and civil engineering labourers, other labourers, cleaners

Table 1

Occupations within social class groupings

Source:
Drever F and Whitehead M (1997)[98]

various assets, and indices based on residential area characteristics. There has been much debate as to what each indicator actually measures, and how choice of indicator influences the pattern of inequalities observed. For example, measures based on occupation may reflect different facets of life for men compared to women, and for people of working age compared to older people or children.

Choice of measure is often dictated by what is available. In Britain occupational social class is frequently used, especially for data collected nationally. Table 1 shows examples of the occupations in each social class group.

Mortality

Over the last twenty years, death rates have fallen among both men and women and across all social groups[25,29]. However, the difference in rates between those at the top and bottom of the social scale has widened.

For example, in the early 1970s, the mortality rate among men of working age was almost twice as high for those in class V (unskilled) as for those in class I (professional). By the early 1990s, it was almost three times higher (table 2). This increasing differential is because, although rates fell overall, they fell more among the high social classes than the low social classes. Between the early 1970s and the early 1990s, rates fell by about 40 per cent for classes I and II, about 30 per cent for classes IIIN, IIIM and IV, but by only 10 per cent for class V. So not only did the differential between the top and the bottom increase, the increase happened across the whole spectrum of social classes[29].

Both class I and class V cover only a small proportion of the population at the extremes of the social scale. Combining class I with class II and class IV with class V allows comparisons of larger sections of the population. Among both men and women aged 35 to 64, overall death rates fell for each group between 1976–81 and 1986–92 (table 3). At the same time, the gap between classes I and II and classes IV and V increased. In the late 1970s, death rates were 53 per cent higher among men in classes IV and V compared with those in classes I and II. In the late 1980s, they were 68 per cent higher. Among women, the differential increased from 50 per cent to 55 per cent[30].

Table 2

European standardised mortality rates, by social class, selected causes, men aged 20–64
England and Wales, selected years

All causes
rates per 100,000

Social class	Year		
	1970–72	1979–83	1991–93
I – Professional	500	373	280
II – Managerial & Technical	526	425	300
III(N) – Skilled (non-manual)	637	522	426
III(M) – Skilled (manual)	683	580	493
IV Partly skilled	721	639	492
V – Unskilled	897	910	806
England and Wales	624	549	419

Lung cancer
rates per 100,000

Social class	Year		
	1970–72	1979–83	1991–93
I – Professional	41	26	17
II – Managerial & Technical	52	39	24
III(N) – Skilled (non-manual)	63	47	34
III(M) – Skilled (manual)	90	72	54
IV Partly skilled	93	76	52
V – Unskilled	109	108	82
England and Wales	73	60	39

Coronary heart disease
rates per 100,000

Social class	Year		
	1970–72	1979–83	1991–93
I – Professional	195	144	81
II – Managerial & Technical	197	168	92
III(N) – Skilled (non-manual)	245	208	136
III(M) – Skilled (manual)	232	218	159
IV – Partly skilled	232	227	156
V – Unskilled	243	287	235
England and Wales	209	201	127

Stroke
rates per 100,000

Social class	Year		
	1970–72	1979–83	1991–93
I – Professional	35	20	14
II – Managerial & Technical	37	23	13
III(N) – Skilled (non-manual)	41	28	19
III(M) – Skilled (manual)	45	34	24
IV – Partly skilled	46	37	25
V – Unskilled	59	55	45
England and Wales	40	30	20

Accidents, poisoning, violence
rates per 100,000

Social class	Year		
	1970–72	1979–83	1991–93
I – Professional	23	17	13
II – Managerial & Technical	25	20	13
III(N) – Skilled (non-manual)	25	21	17
III(M) – Skilled (manual)	34	27	24
IV – Partly skilled	39	35	24
V – Unskilled	67	63	52
England and Wales	34	28	22

Suicide and undetermined injury
rates per 100,000

Social class	Year		
	1970–72	1979–83	1991–93
I – Professional	16	16	13
II – Managerial & Technical	13	15	14
III(N) – Skilled (non-manual)	17	18	20
III(M) – Skilled (manual)	12	16	21
IV – Partly skilled	18	23	23
V – Unskilled	32	44	47
England and Wales	15	20	22

Source: Drever F, Bunting J (1997)[29]

Table 3		Women (35–64)			Men (35–64)		
		1976–81	1981–85	1986–92	1976–81	1981–85	1986–92
Age-standardised mortality rates per 100,000 people, by social class, selected causes, men and women aged 35–64, England and Wales, 1976–92	**All causes**						
	I/II	338	344	270	621	539	455
	IIIN	371	387	305	860	658	484
	IIIM	467	396	356	802	691	624
Source: Harding S, Bethune A, Maxwell R, Brown J (1997)[30]	IV/V	508	445	418	951	824	764
	Ratio IV/V:I/II	1.50	1.29	1.55	1.53	1.53	1.68
	Coronary heart disease						
	I/II	39	45	29	246	185	160
	IIIN	56	57	39	382	267	162
	IIIM	85	67	59	309	269	231
	IV/V	105	76	78	363	293	266
	Ratio IV/V:I/II	2.69	1.69	2.69	1.48	1.58	1.66
	Breast cancer						
	I/II	52	74	52			
	IIIN	75	71	49			
	IIIM	61	57	46			
	IV/V	47	50	54			
	Ratio IV/V:I/II	0.90	0.68	1.04			

These growing differences across the social spectrum were apparent for many of the major causes of death, including coronary heart disease, stroke, lung cancer and suicides among men, and respiratory disease and lung cancer among women[29,30].

Death rates can be summarised into average life expectancy at birth. For men in classes I and II combined, life expectancy increased by 2 years between the late 1970s and the late 1980s. For those in classes IV and V combined, the increase was smaller, 1.4 years. The difference between those at the top and bottom of the social class scale in the late 1980s was 5 years, 75 years compared with 70 years. For women, the differential was smaller, 80 years compared with 77 years. Improvements in life expectancy have been greater over the period from the late 1970s to the late 1980s for women in classes I and II than for those in classes IV and V, two years compared to one year[31].

A good measure of inequality among older people is life expectancy at age 65. Again, in the late 1980s, this was considerably higher among those in higher social classes, and the differential increased over the period from the late 1970s to the late 1980s, particularly for women[31].

Table 4		Numbers of lives lost	Working man-years lost	Proportion of deaths from these diseases
Estimates of the numbers of lives and working man-years lost per year, selected causes, men aged 20–64, England and Wales, 1991–93	Coronary heart disease	5,000	47,000	28%
	Accidents etc	1,500	41,000	43%
	Suicide etc	1,300	39,000	40%
Note: Estimates assume all men have mortality rates as for social class I and II. Only deaths at ages 20–64 years are included in the analysis	Lung cancer	2,300	16,500	42%
	Other neoplasms	1,700	21,000	13%
	Respiratory disease	1,500	12,500	47%
Source: Drever F. Unpublished analysis (1998)	Stroke	900	9,000	32%
	All diseases	**17,200**	**240,000**	**29%**

Years of life lost

Premature mortality, that is death before age 65, is higher among people who are unskilled. Table 4 illustrates this with an analysis of deaths in men aged 20 to 64 years. If all men in this age group had the same death rates as those in classes I and II, it is estimated that there would have been over 17,000 fewer deaths each year from 1991 to 1993. Deaths from accidents and suicide occur at relatively young ages and each contribute nearly as much to overall years of working life lost as coronary heart disease. Death rates from all three causes are higher among those in the lower social classes, and markedly so among those in class V[32,33].

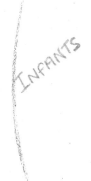

These major differences in death rates and life expectancy between social classes do not just apply to those people already well into adulthood. Infant mortality rates are also lower among babies born to those of higher social classes. In 1994–96, nearly 5 out of every thousand babies born to parents in class I and II died in their first year. For those babies born in to families in classes IV and V, the infant mortality rate was over 7 per thousand babies. As with mortality at other ages, infant mortality rates in each class have been decreasing over the last twenty years. However, there is no evidence that the class differential in infant mortality has decreased over this period[34].

Morbidity

Although death rates have fallen and life expectancy increased, there is little evidence that the population is experiencing less morbidity or disability than 10 or 20 years ago. There has been a slight increase in self-reported long standing illness and limiting long standing illness, and socioeconomic differences are substantial. For example, in 1996 among the 45 to 64 age group, 17 per cent of professional men reported a limiting long standing illness compared to 48 per cent of unskilled men. Among women, 25 per cent of professional women and 45 per cent of unskilled women reported such a condition. These patterns were similar among younger adults, older men and among children[28].

OBESITY

In adulthood, being overweight is a measure of possible ill health, with obesity a risk factor for many chronic diseases. There is a marked social class gradient in obesity which is greater among women than among men[35][37]. In 1996, 25 per cent of women in class V were classified as obese compared to 14 per cent of women in class I. For men, there was no clear difference in the proportions reported as obese except that men in class I had lower rates of obesity, 11 per cent, compared to about 18 per cent in other groups. Overall, rates of obesity are rising. For men, 13 per cent were classified as obese in 1993 compared to 16 per cent in 1996. For women, the rise was from 16 per cent to 18 per cent[37].

HYPERTENSION

Another indicator of poor health is raised blood pressure. There is a clear social class differential among women, with those in higher classes being less likely than those in the manual classes to have hypertension. In 1996, 17 per cent of women in class I and 24 per cent in class V had hypertension. There was no such difference for men where the comparable proportions were 20 per cent and 21 per cent respectively[37].

ACCIDENTS

Among men, major accidents are more common in the manual classes for those aged under 55. Between 55 and 64, the non-manual classes have higher major accident rates (figure 3). For women, there are no differences in accident rates until after the age of 75 when those women in the non-manual group have higher rates of major accidents[37].

Figure 3

Annual major accident rates, by age and social class, England 1996

Source:
Prescott-Clarke P, Primatesta P (1998)[37]

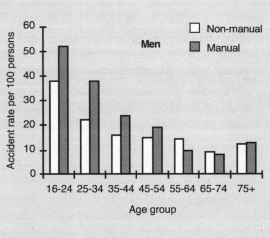

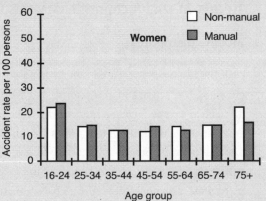

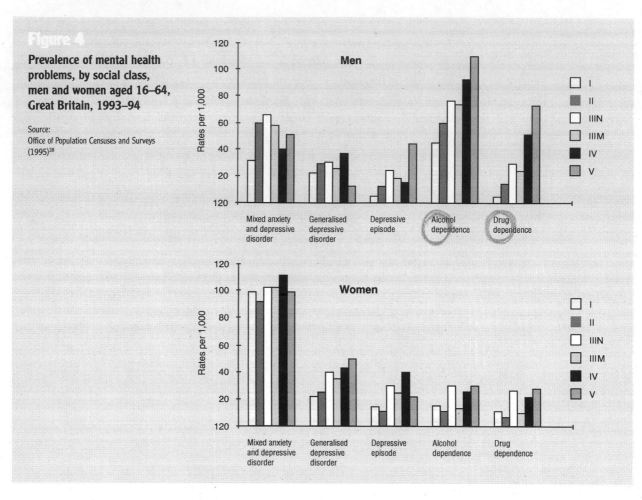

Figure 4

Prevalence of mental health problems, by social class, men and women aged 16–64, Great Britain, 1993–94

Source:
Office of Population Censuses and Surveys (1995)[38]

Mental health also varies markedly by social class. In 1993/4, all neurotic disorders, such as anxiety, depression and phobias, were more common among women in class IV and V than those in classes I and II – 24 per cent and 15 per cent respectively[38]. This difference was not seen among men. However, there were striking gradients for alcohol and drug dependence among men, but not women. For example, 10 per cent of men in classes IV and V were dependent on alcohol compared to 5 per cent in classes I and II, (figure 4)[38].

Trends in socioeconomic determinants of health

Income distribution

Over the last twenty years, household disposable income per head of population has grown both in actual and in real terms. Between 1961 and 1994, average household disposable income (in real terms) rose by 72 per cent[39]. However, this was not experienced to the same extent across the whole of the income distribution.
The median real household disposable income, before housing costs, rose over the period 1961 to 1994 from £136 per week, to £234 per week (figure 5). The top decile point more than doubled, from £233 per week to £473 per week. The bottom decile point rose by 62 per cent from £74 per week to £119 per week.

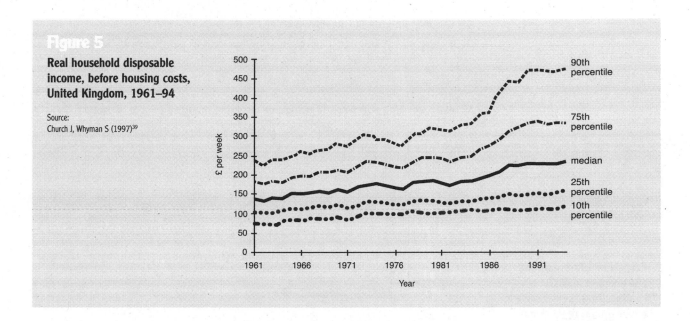

Figure 5

Real household disposable income, before housing costs, United Kingdom, 1961–94

Source:
Church J, Whyman S (1997)[39]

Households below average income

The proportion of people whose income is below average has been at about 60 per cent for the last 35 years (figure 6). However, the proportion of people below half of the average income (the European Union definition of poverty) has grown over this period from 10 per cent in 1961 to 20 per cent in 1991. It has decreased since then and was at 17 per cent in 1995[40].

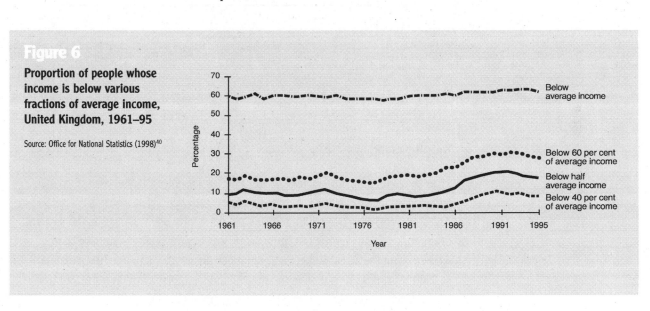

Figure 6

Proportion of people whose income is below various fractions of average income, United Kingdom, 1961–95

Source: Office for National Statistics (1998)[40]

Education

Since the early 1970s, the proportion of children aged 3 or 4 who attend school has trebled from 20 per cent to nearly 60 per cent[40]. The proportion who attend school (as opposed to playgroups) varies from 84 per cent in the North East to 43 per cent in the South West[41].

Educational attainment – as measured by the proportion of children gaining 5 or more GCSEs at grades A star to C – has risen from less than 25 per cent in 1975/76 to about 45 per cent in 1995/96[40,42]. This measure of attainment varies not only by gender, but also by geographical area and by measures of deprivation.

As well as looking at the future workforce and their qualifications, it is useful to look at the educational attainment of those presently of working age[40]. In 1997, 16 per cent of men and 21 per cent of women of working age had no qualifications. There were also large differences between ethnic groups (figure 7).

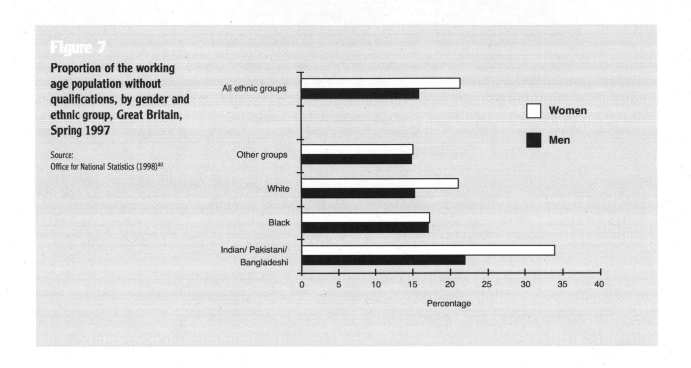

Figure 7

Proportion of the working age population without qualifications, by gender and ethnic group, Great Britain, Spring 1997

Source:
Office for National Statistics (1998)[40]

Employment

The seasonally adjusted unemployment rate for those aged 16 and over stood at 6.2 per cent in summer 1998, almost three times the level of 30 years ago[43]. Although rates have been falling since 1993, there have been changes in the patterns of unemployment over the last thirty years, well beyond what might have been expected from seasonal and cyclical variations (figure 8). Youth unemployment is still at higher rates now than it was in 1991 and unemployment rates are four times higher among unskilled workers than among professional groups[44].

Across different ethnic groups, there are very different rates of unemployment (table 5). Those from minority ethnic groups have higher rates than the white population. Black men have particularly high unemployment rates as do Pakistani and Bangladeshi women[45].

Figure 8

Unemployment rates, population aged 16 years and over, England and Wales, 1961–1995

Source:
Church J, Whyman S (1997)[39]

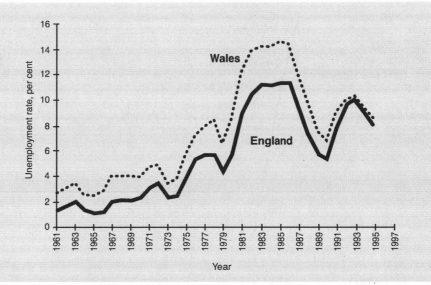

Table 5

Unemployment rates, by ethnic group, Great Britain, winter 1997/98

Note:
Sample size is too small to make accurate estimates of unemployment rates amongst Chinese people.

Source:
Office for National Statistics (1998)[45]

	Percentage	
	Men	Women
White	6.5	5.0
All minority ethnic groups	14.1	13.1
Black	20.5	14.8
Indian	7.4	8.4
Pakistani/Bangladeshi	15.9	22.1
Other	15	14

Housing

Over the last sixty years, the number of dwellings has doubled from 10.6 million in 1938 to 20.7 million in 1997[46,47]. Housing tenure has also changed dramatically over this period with a doubling of the proportion of owner-occupied dwellings[46,47] and a dramatic fall in the proportion of privately rented dwellings (table 6).

There has also been a growth in the number of one-person households over the last ten years from 4.4 million in 1984 to 5.5 million in 1995/96[48]. The proportion of all

Table 6

Proportion of dwellings by household tenure, England, 1938 and 1997

Source:
Department of the Environment, Transport and the Regions (1998)[47]

	Percentage	
	1938	1997
Owner occupied	32	68
Local authority or New Town rented	11	17
Housing association rented	n/a	5
Privately rented	57	10
Number of dwellings	10.6 million	20.7 million

Table 7

Household tenure, one person households, England, 1984 and 1995/6

Source:
Office for National Statistics (1997)[48]

	Thousands	
	1984	1995/96
Owner occupiers	2,008	2,923
Social rented sector	1,657	1,771
Private rented sector	746	760
All tenures	4,410	5,453

households which had only one person rose from 25 per cent to 28 per cent over this period. In 1984, 46 per cent of one-person households were owner occupied. By 1995/96, this had grown to 54 per cent (table 7).

Between 1991 and 2016, the number of households is expected to rise from 19.2 million to 23.6 million – a rise of 4.4 million households[49].

Conditions of the housing stock vary considerably. In 1996 about 14 per cent of all households were living in poor conditions. About 8 per cent of dwellings in England were unfit, and about 7 per cent of households were living in unfit dwellings. The proportions of households in unfit dwellings varied with the type of tenure, from 4 per cent in the Registered Social Landlord sector to 18 per cent of households who rented from private landlords. In urban areas, 8 per cent of dwellings were deemed unfit whereas in rural areas, 5 per cent were deemed unfit[50].

Homelessness

Between 1982 and 1992, there was a steep increase in the number of households accepted by Local Authorities as homeless. Since then, there has been a decrease of about a quarter. Of the 166,000 households classified as homeless in 1997, over 103,000 were accepted by local authorities to be unintentionally homeless and in priority need. Over half of households accepted by local authorities as homeless had dependent children and a further tenth had a pregnant household member[51].

Public safety

The crime rate has nearly trebled since 1971. In 1996, the crime rate in England was nearly one crime for every ten people[40]. Crime rates were highest in areas with large conurbations – the North East, Yorkshire/Humberside and London[41]. There were also different crime rates in different types of areas – lowest in affluent suburban and rural areas and highest in council estates and low income areas (table 8).

Different areas of the country have very different rates of particular types of crime. London has the highest rate of fraud and forgery, robbery and sexual offences. The North East has the highest rate of criminal damage and the lowest rate of sexual offences. Yorkshire and the Humber has the highest burglary rate. The East has the lowest overall crime rate[41].

Table 8

Risk of being a victim of crime, by type of area, England and Wales, 1995

Percentage

	Council estates and low income	Affluent family	Affluent urban	New home-owning	Mature home-owning	Affluent suburban and rural
Thefts of vehicles	25	21	21	21	18	16
Vandalism of vehicles	11	7	12	10	8	6
Bicycle thefts	10	3	8	8	5	3
Burglary	10	4	8	6	6	4
Home vandalism	5	5	5	5	4	3
Other household theft	9	7	8	8	7	5
Any household offence	36	35	35	33	31	27

Source: Office for National Statistics (1998)[40]

Transport

Access to private means of transport has increased in recent years. In 1996, 70 per cent of households had access to a car or a van. This compared with just over half of households in 1972. About a quarter of households had access to two or more cars and vans compared to only 9 per cent in 1972 (figure 9)[28,52,53].

Those with access to two or more cars or vans were not only more likely to be economically active, but also tended to be in the higher socioeconomic groups. Only seven per cent of households had access to two or more vehicles when the head of

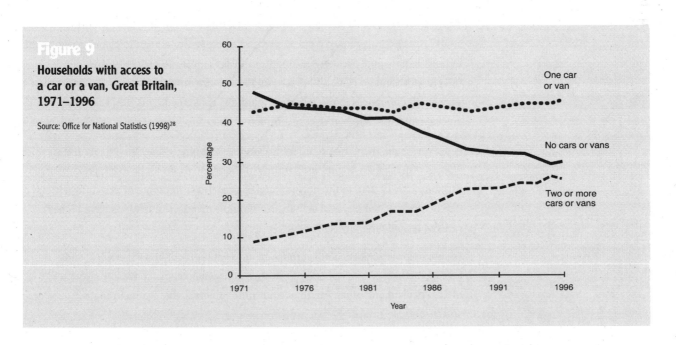

Figure 9

Households with access to a car or a van, Great Britain, 1971–1996

Source: Office for National Statistics (1998)[28]

household was economically inactive compared to 36 per cent of households with an economically active head[28]. In 1991, those who lived in the social rented sector had the highest proportion with no access to a car, 68 per cent, while those in the owner occupied sector had the smallest proportion with no access, 19 per cent[52].

How people travel to work differs depending on whether the areas in which they live are urban or rural[54]. In England in 1991, 60 per cent of people travelled to work by car in urban areas and 69 per cent in rural areas. Rail and bus accounted for 17 per cent of journeys to work for those in urban areas but only for five per cent for rural areas. A higher proportion of people work at home in rural areas, 12 per cent compared to four per cent in urban areas (table 9).

Table 9

Mode of travel to work, England, 1991

Source:
Office for National Statistics (1997)[54]

	Percentage	
	Urban	Rural
Car	60	69
Rail or bus	17	5
On foot	12	7
By pedal cycle	3	2
Work at home	4	12

Health related behaviour

Over the last twenty years, the proportion of people who report that they smoke cigarettes has fallen. In 1974, roughly a half of men and two fifths of women smoked cigarettes, compared with less than 30 per cent of men and women in 1996. The trends in drinking alcohol are broadly unchanged over this period. However, the proportion of women who drank more than 14 units of alcohol a week rose from 9 per cent in 1984 to 14 per cent in 1996[28].

There is a clear social class gradient for both men and women in the proportion who smoke. In 1996, this ranged from 12 per cent of professional men to 41 per cent of men in unskilled manual occupations and from 11 per cent to 36 per cent for women[28]. In spite of the major class differences in dependence on alcohol in men[38], there are very small differences in the reported quantities consumed. This is not the case among women where higher consumption is related to higher social class[28].

Among women, there are no differences in levels of physical activity across the social classes. Among men, higher proportions in the manual classes have a high level of physical activity than in the non-manual classes. However, some of this difference is due to work related physical activity. Men in non-manual occupations have higher rates of leisure time physical activity[35].

People in lower socioeconomic groups tend to eat less fruit and vegetables, and less food which is rich in dietary fibre. As a consequence, they have lower intakes of anti-oxidant and other vitamins, and some minerals, than those in higher socioeconomic groups[35,55–58].

One aspect of dietary behaviour that affects the health of infants is the incidence of breastfeeding. Six weeks after birth, almost three quarters of babies in class I households are still breastfed. This declines with class to less than one quarter of babies in class V. The differences between classes in rates of breastfeeding at six weeks has narrowed slightly between 1985 and 1995[59].

Trends in health differences between minority ethnic groups

There are many indications of poorer health among the minority ethnic groups in England. For example, people in Black (Caribbean, African and other) groups and Indians have higher rates of limiting long standing illness than white people. Those of Pakistani or Bangladeshi origin have the highest rates. In contrast, the Chinese and "other Asians" have rates lower than the white population[60].

Although in analysing mortality rates we have to use country of birth as a proxy for ethnicity, a similar pattern emerges[61]. There is excess mortality among men and women born in Africa and men born on the Indian sub-continent and men and women born in Scotland or Ireland (table 10).

Table 10

Standardised mortality ratios, by country of birth, selected causes, men and women aged 20–69, England and Wales, 1989–92

	All causes		Coronary heart disease		Stroke		Lung cancer		Breast cancer
	Men	Women	Men	Women	Men	Women	Men	Women	Women
All countries	100	100	100	100	100	100	100	100	100
Scotland	132	136	120	130	125	125	149	169	114
Ireland	139	120	124	120	138	123	151	147	92
East Africa	110	103	131	105	114	122	42	17	84
West Africa	113	126	56	62	271	181	62	51	125
Caribbean	77	91	46	71	168	157	49	31	75
South Asia	106	100	146	151	155	141	45	33	59

Source: Wild S, McKeigue P (1997)[61]

This table was first published in the British Medical Journal, and is reproduced by kind permission of the journal.

Many women from minority ethnic groups giving birth in the 1990s were born in the United Kingdom. Because country of birth of the mother, and not ethnicity, is recorded at birth registration, it is not possible to estimate infant mortality rates by minority ethnic group. However, among mothers who were born in countries outside the UK, those from the Caribbean and Pakistan have infant mortality rates about double the national average. Perinatal mortality rates have also been consistently higher for babies of mothers born outside the UK. The differences between groups have not decreased over the last twenty years[34].

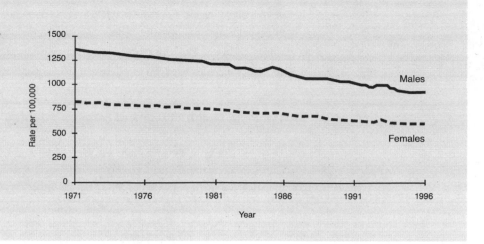

Figure 10

Standardised mortality rates, by gender, all ages, England and Wales, 1971–96

Source:
Office for National Statistics (1998)[25]

Trends in health differences between the sexes

Death rates have been falling for both males and for females (figure 10). Since 1971, these have decreased by 29 per cent for males and by 25 per cent for females, narrowing the differential in death rates very slightly. Cancers and coronary heart disease account for 55 per cent of the deaths of men and 42 per cent of the deaths of women[25].

At each age in childhood, and on into adulthood, the age-specific mortality rates for boys is higher than for girls (figure 11)[62]. For the under 5s, nearly half of the difference is due to external causes, in particular accidental drowning and submersion. For children aged 5 to 14, external causes, chiefly motor vehicle traffic accidents, account for nearly 70 per cent of the difference[25].

Although the life expectancy gap between males and females is decreasing[26], this is not the case for healthy life expectancy. Healthy life expectancy of females is only

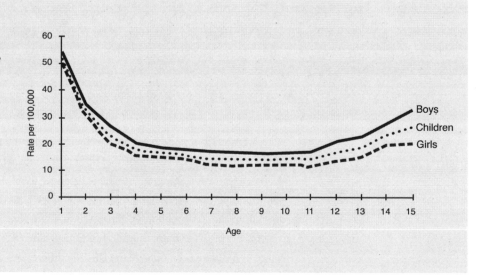

Figure 11

Age-specific mortality rates, children, England and Wales, 1991–1995

Source:
Botting B (1997)[62]

Figure 12

Prevalence of major accidents, by gender and age, England, 1996

Source:
Prescott-Clarke P, Primatesta P (1998)[37]

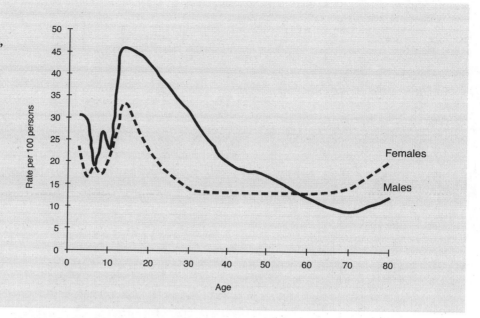

two to three years more than that of males[27]. Overall, there is little difference in the proportions of males and females reporting a limiting long standing illness[53]. Women report more illness of many different types than men during the reproductive years[53].

For both children and adults of working ages, males have higher major accident rates than females (figure 12). At older ages, women have higher major accident rates than men[37].

The proportion of smokers is higher among girls than boys[63]. By adulthood, the proportions of men and women smoking are about the same (29 and 28 per cent), compared with 51 per cent of men and 41 per cent of women in 1974[53]. For both children and adults, males are more likely to drink alcohol heavily than females[53].

Conclusion

(Inequalities by socioeconomic group, ethnic group and gender can be demonstrated across a wide range of measures of health and the determinants of health. Analysis of these patterns and trends in inequalities has informed the development of areas for future policy development) which are considered in Part 2.

PART 2

Reducing Inequalities in Health

Introduction: assessing the evidence

We have sought to ensure that our recommendations are based on scientific and expert evidence. To this end, we have consulted with a wide range of experts and incorporated a process of peer review. In summary, we commissioned a series of input papers from experts broadly to match the sections of the report. Most of these experts consulted widely amongst other researchers in their field. For each of these commissioned papers, we obtained an independent scientific commentary. We also sought and received a considerable volume of material from institutions and individuals with expertise or experience relevant to inequalities in health, including scientific reviews and papers. A separate Evaluation Group was convened to consider the commissioned papers with associated commentaries and asked to report on the quality of the evidence on which the recommendations in the papers were based, and to identify gaps[64]. A more detailed description of the process is given in annex B.

All this material was considered and discussed within the Scientific Advisory Group. The material reflected a wealth of descriptive data documenting inequalities in health and a growing quantity of research exploring mechanisms. However, controlled intervention studies are rare. Indeed, the more a potential intervention relates to the wider determinants of inequalities in health (ie "upstream" policies), the less the possibility of using the methodology of a controlled trial to evaluate it. We have, therefore evaluated many different types of evidence in forming our judgement. The following sections incorporate our assessment of the full spectrum of evidence which we reviewed.

Cross-Government Issues

If future inequalities in health are to be reduced, it will be essential to carry out a wide range of policies to achieve both a general improvement in health and a greater impact on the less well off. By this we mean those who in terms of socioeconomic status, gender or ethnicity are less well off than average in terms of health or its principal determinants – such as income, education, employment or the material environment.

The impact of policies designed to improve health may have different consequences for different groups of people which are not always appreciated. Some policies will both improve health and reduce health inequalities. The introduction of the NHS benefited the health of all sections of the population, particularly women and children, many of whom were excluded from previous arrangements under the National Insurance Act.

A well intended policy which improves average health may have no effect on inequalities. It may even widen them by having a greater impact on the better off. Classic examples include policies aimed at preventing illness, if they resulted in uptake favouring the better off. This has happened in some initiatives concerned with immunisation and cervical screening, as well as in some campaigns to discourage smoking or to promote breastfeeding. More recently, the Government's welcome decision to provide a pre-school place for every child aged four in the country is likely to benefit health on average but could have the unintended effect of increasing inequalities. This would happen if the children of the better off made more effective use of the service.

These examples highlight the need for extra attention to the needs of the less well off. This could be accommodated both by policies directed at the least well off and by an approach which would require the need for inequalities to be addressed wherever universal services are provided, such as publicly funded education and the National Health Service, and where other policies are likely to have an impact on health.

A broader approach of this kind which explicitly addresses inequalities could provide a new direction for public policy. It is our view that, in general, reductions in inequalities are most likely to be achieved if policies are formulated with the reduction of inequalities in mind.

1. We RECOMMEND that as part of health impact assessment, all policies likely to have a direct or indirect effect on health should be evaluated in terms of their impact on health inequalities, and should be formulated in such a way that by favouring the less well off they will, wherever possible, reduce such inequalities.

This proposal for a systematic impact assessment of policy on health inequalities is a significant extension to the steps already taken by Government to apply impact assessments to its policies[1], and to ensure better coordination across Whitehall.

We suggest that this proposal needs to be supported by a small and effective unit with a pan-Government view. Such a lead by Government would allow action on inequalities to be both reviewed and promoted. It would also serve to further encourage the steps being taken to strengthen coordination at both central and local level.

1.1 We recommend establishing mechanisms to monitor inequalities in health and to evaluate the effectiveness of measures taken to reduce them.

The effects of future policies will need to be monitored at regular intervals. For this purpose, the Government will require authoritative statistics on inequalities in health and the factors influencing them at national and local level. These will also be needed in order to set targets for reduction of health inequalities. A number of concerns about the presently available data have been raised with us. These include the scope for monitoring inequalities among older people, when many data sources have an effective cut-off point of age 64. There are continuing inconsistencies in the treatment of males and females in the census and at death registration, where married women are still mainly classified by the social class of their husband. There is also a need for greater consistency between data from the census, from vital registration and from other sources.

1.2 *We recommend a review of data needs to improve the capacity to monitor inequalities in health and their determinants at a national and local level.*

We have emphasised the priority we will be giving to parents and children in the report as the best way of reducing future inequalities in physical and mental health. This issue is relevant across Government.

2. *We RECOMMEND a high priority is given to policies aimed at improving health and reducing health inequalities in women of childbearing age, expectant mothers and young children.*

Areas for Future Policy Development

1. Poverty, Income, Tax and Benefits

Poverty and income

Inequality

Inequalities in health are of long standing and their determinants are deeply ingrained in our social structure. Since 1980, although health and expectation of life have generally improved, the social gradients of many indicators of health have deteriorated or at best remained unchanged. Although this period was also marked by substantial economic growth, income differentials widened to a degree not seen since the Second World War. It also saw the reversal in the trend to greater equality seen in the 1960s and 1970s. Average incomes grew in real terms by about 40 per cent between 1979 and 1994/5, but this growth was far greater (60–68 per cent) amongst the richest tenth of the population. For the poorest tenth average income increased by only 10 per cent (before housing costs) or fell by 8 per cent (after them). There has been some improvement in the relative position of the poorest groups in the period since 1992 but income inequality is still pronounced and is worse than in many other developed countries[65].

The differences in incomes between those on means-tested benefits and those with other sources of income are a major determinant of income inequality in the United Kingdom. Among the poorest fifth of the population, the majority have incomes set by the level of means-tested benefit[65]. People on low income, defined as below half average income, are more likely to be unemployed, lone parents and their children, people with disabilities or pensioners and to live in social housing. Some minority ethnic groups, especially Pakistanis and Bangladeshis, are over-represented in the poorest fifth of the income distribution[65-69].

A similar picture emerges if poverty is defined as the receipt of Income Support. Almost a quarter of all households include at least one person receiving Income Support[70]. Measured over a two year period, this figure rises to more than a third. The number of people receiving Income Support has risen from just over 4 million in 1979 to 9.6 million in 1996[71]. Comparisons over time are difficult but recent work has shown that the proportion of the population with below half average income has more than doubled since 1979, to reach 18 per cent in the mid 1990s[72].

Many studies and analyses have demonstrated the association of increasingly poor health with increasing material disadvantage. For instance, all cause mortality is correlated with Townsend deprivation score, an index which combines indicators of unemployment, lack of car, not being an owner occupier and overcrowding. The highest mortality rates for both men and women are found among those who live in areas with the highest scores (most deprived), and the lowest in those from areas which are least deprived[73]. People living in households with incomes of £350 or more per week have significantly lower rates of self-reported long standing illness than those living in households with an income of £200 per week or less[74]. However, available evidence is insufficient to confirm or deny a causal relationship between changes in income distribution and the parallel deterioration in inequalities in some areas of ill health. Nevertheless, we take the view that these changes are likely to be related. In addition to being responsible for part of the burden of morbidity and mortality, they probably contribute to the persistence of the steep, unfavourable socioeconomic gradients in smoking and in the consumption of important nutrients such as antioxidants. Perhaps even more important is the damage persistent family and childhood poverty does to the health of future generations.

We welcome the Government's declared intention to redress income inequalities through the establishment of a national minimum wage, "Welfare to Work" and other measures. This approach should be accompanied by efforts to redistribute resources, in cash or kind, to those who, for reasons such as age or disability, are unable to work, and to those families for whom work is not available or appropriate. We consider that without a shift of resources to the less well off, both in and out of work, little will be accomplished in terms of a reduction of health inequalities by interventions addressing particular "downstream" influences.

Tax and Benefits

A fairer tax system will help the less well-off who are in work. It can boost the incomes of those in low paid work, neutralise the poverty trap for those able to work and reduce inequalities. Recent changes, such as "Welfare to Work" and the announcement of the Working Families Tax Credit Scheme in the 1998 Budget, explicitly recognise the link between tax and benefits for working families. It is too early to assess the effects of these changes and they will need to be kept under review. It is our view that more may need to be done. Over the last 20 years a greater proportion of total taxation has been raised by indirect taxes[75], notably through VAT but also through excise duties. We note the Government's pledge not to extend VAT to food, children's clothes and public transport fares, and the action it has taken to reduce VAT on domestic fuels in a direct effort to help poorer and older people. Shifting the tax burden from regressive to more progressive forms of taxation and fiscal policies which take account of the combined impact of direct and indirect taxation on the living standards of lower income groups, would help mitigate the effects of income inequalities.

For the least well-off members of society, however, it is the benefit system which is the principal determinant of living standards. A comprehensive review of the social security system and its implications for health are beyond the capacity and competence of the Inquiry. Welfare reform is, however, on the Government's agenda. We believe it is important that, over time, benefit and pensions levels are set at a level sufficient to pay for items and services necessary for health and for participation in society.

We have decided to focus on two groups where we believe the current system fosters major inequalities in health and which will not reap the full benefits of the Government's recent, work-related reforms. These groups are families with children and pensioners.

Evidence

Poverty falls disproportionately on children. In the mid 1990s, around one in four of the total population in Britain were living in poverty (below 50% of average income after housing costs). Among children, the proportion was one in three[76]. In 1996, 2.2 million children were in a family receiving Income Support[77].

A child, and additional children, has a much greater impact on the standard of living of poorer than better-off households[78]. Yet current levels of benefits are not generous, either relative to average incomes or to levels found in much of continental Europe[79]. Income Support falls significantly short of the level that independent experts determine to be the modern minimum. In 1992/3, the income of a single pensioner, owner occupier on Income Support fell £8 per week short of the standard; a couple with two children needed £34 more benefit to reach the standard[80,81]. Depending on age, Income Support rates meet between 67 per cent and 90 per cent of minimum needs of children, as assessed by a representative cross-section of parents[82]. Another study found that Income Support levels are insufficient to meet the costs of an adequate diet for expectant mothers, particularly single women under the age of 25[83]. Studies of the cost of meeting the basic needs of children of different ages suggest not only that the income provided by Income Support is insufficient but that the personal allowances for children understate the costs of younger children (especially those under 2 years) relative to older children[65,84]. Independent and expert assessment of basic needs also indicates that the personal allowances paid to one- and two-parent families underestimate the relative cost of providing a basic standard of living for one-parent families[78,84,85]. It is estimated that a lone parent with two children would need 93% of the amount required by a couple with two children to achieve the same "modest but adequate" standard of living[85]. The 1998 Budget with above inflation increases in the benefit rates for younger children, childcare tax credit for working parents and the working families tax credit will contribute to the narrowing of these discrepancies. Substantial improvement will require sustained action but this is an important start which goes some way to narrowing these discrepancies but will not eliminate them.

The switch to link benefits to prices rather than earnings in the early 1980s has meant a relative deterioration in the position of groups who rely on benefits, including pensioners (figure 13)[65]. The poorest pensioners are those wholly dependent on the State Retirement pension and although this is designed to be supplemented by Income

Support, some one million – or around one in four of state retirement pensioners – do not claim support to which they are entitled[86,87]. A number of factors may operate, including lack of knowledge of entitlement, a perception of being stigmatised by the receipt of benefit and physical or other difficulties in the processes of claiming. Possible ways of overcoming some of these problems are the establishment of new organisations or agencies: a pensioner's agency as a way of achieving "one-stop" provision of welfare[88]: a citizen's bank[88]: or a welfare "counsellor" in primary care centres in disadvantaged areas[89,90]. A further suggestion to the Inquiry has been that an Income Support "top-up" could be paid automatically to bring the poorest pensioners up to Income Support levels.

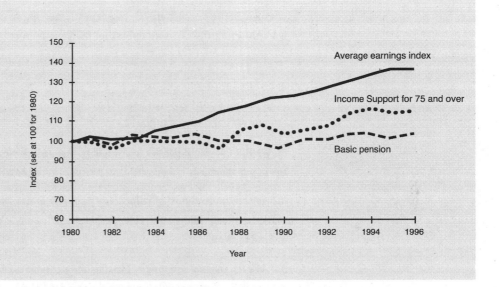

Figure 13

Indices of average earnings, basic pensions and Income Support for those aged 75 and over, United Kingdom, 1980–1996

Source:
Centre for Analysis of Social Exclusion, London School of Economics, unpublished (1998)

There is a lack of experimental evidence that increasing financial resources results in measurable health gain. A rare exception is a randomised controlled trial carried out in Gary, Indiana, USA between 1970 and 1974. The intervention group received an expanded income support plan which guaranteed a minimum income to a group of mothers with low income. Mothers at high risk of adverse pregnancy outcome had heavier babies if they had received the income support plan[91]. However a review, which is being carried out under the auspices of the Cochrane Collaboration, has not been able to identify other evaluations of financial support interventions which include health outcomes, meeting review quality criteria[64].

Thus the bulk of the empirical evidence comes from research demonstrating that people living on low incomes, including those whose income consists entirely of state benefits, have insufficient money to buy items and services necessary for good health. Studies of the budgeting arrangements of poor families show that the money for food is often used as the reserve to iron out fluctuations in income and meet emergencies[92]. Mothers often shop alone to curtail expenditure and shop frequently to prevent food being available at home and therefore at risk of being consumed before it is essential. Spending is much reduced in the second week of the benefit cycle. Families can and do go short of food during this time because of shortage of money and, more often than not, it is the mother who goes without[93–95]. Some mothers have nutritionally deficient diets, although they are usually successful in protecting the diets of their children[94]. Older people are particularly at risk of "fuel poverty" and may under-heat their homes because they cannot afford to buy fuel[96,97]. Poverty may also act as a barrier for older people to services and care and to an adequate diet.

Benefit

Policies which increase the income of the poorest are likely to improve their living standards, such as nutrition and heating and so lead to improvements in health. This can be done by improving social security benefits, specifically for families with young children and pensioners, by increasing employment opportunities and through changes in the tax system. We have already noted that what is affordable in this area is a matter for the Government rather than the Inquiry.

At a population level, improvements in income and living standards are clearly associated with improvements in health and life expectancy[98]. As the effects of such interventions on individual health have not been tested, any possible harmful side effects are unknown, if unlikely.

3. We RECOMMEND policies which will further reduce income inequalities, and improve the living standards of households in receipt of social security benefits. Specifically:

3.1 we recommend further reductions in poverty in women of childbearing age, expectant mothers, young children and older people should be made by increasing benefits in cash or in kind to them.

3.2 We recommend uprating of benefits and pensions according to principles which protect and, where possible, improve the standard of living of those who depend on them, and which narrow the gap between their standard of living and average living standards.

3.3 We recommend measures to increase the uptake of benefits in entitled groups.

We recommend further steps to increase employment opportunities (recommendation 8.1).

2. Education

Education plays a number of roles in influencing inequalities in health, if health is viewed in its widest sense. Firstly, it has an important role in influencing inequalities in socioeconomic position. Educational qualifications are a determinant of an individual's labour market position, which in turn influences income, housing and other material resources. These are related to health and health inequalities. As a consequence, education is a traditional route out of poverty for those living in disadvantage.

Secondly, education has a role in preparing children for life, in particular in ensuring that they have the practical, social and emotional knowledge and skills to achieve a full and healthy life. These include knowledge of the wider determinants of health, not just health related behaviour, skills in developing relationships and dealing with conflict, and practical skills such as budgeting and cooking.

Thirdly, education has a social role in preparing children to participate fully in society. This includes making children aware of their democratic rights and responsibilities, educating them about using services, co-operation and working together and enhancing greater understanding of other groups in society. The role of the school as part of the local community is an important component in achieving these outcomes.

Fourthly, the education system should protect and promote the current health of children, by providing an environment and culture which is safe, healthy and conducive to learning[99–101].

We recognise that a group of children at particular disadvantage are those who are excluded from school or who are frequent truants. These children and young people include disproportionate numbers with special educational needs, from minority ethnic groups, and who are looked-after by local authorities. School exclusion and truancy are associated with increased involvement in crime, as victims and perpetrators, substance misuse and other dangerous activities. In the long term, school exclusion and truancy are associated with unemployment, imprisonment, homelessness and teenage pregnancy. Measures to enable local education authorities to reduce truancy and exclusion are essential if the educational opportunities of this vulnerable group of children are to be protected. We note the recent report from the Government's Social Exclusion Unit on this topic. In view of its special recommendations to education and other authorities, we have not made recommendations in this area. We believe that the policy areas we recommend in this report which support parents and children at home and school will address the "upstream" factors which lead to exclusion and truancy. These policy areas should complement those recommended in the Social Exclusion Unit's report[102].

This section is based on the recognition of the roles of education in reducing inequalities in health. Our recommendations in this area relate to increasing the resources for schools serving the less well off, further development of pre-school education and health promoting schools and improving nutrition at school.

Increasing resources for schools serving the less well off

Inequality

The roles of education set out above imply a range of outcomes which are not readily measurable. However, inequality is observed when looking at educational achievement. Children from disadvantaged backgrounds, as measured by being in receipt of free school meals, have lower educational achievement than other children. Local education authorities (LEAs) with a high percentage of pupils eligible for free school meals (an indicator of poverty) have a low percentage of pupils with 5 or more passes at GCSE levels A star to C (figure 14). Higher proportions of pupils in the south of England gain 5 or more passes at GCSE grades A star to C than in the north-east[41].

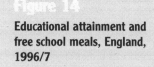

Figure 14

Educational attainment and free school meals, England, 1996/7

Source:
Hansard (1998) 307;801–805

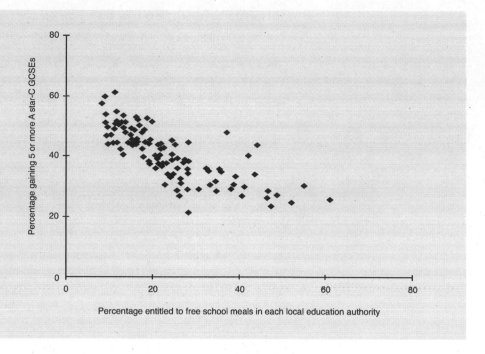

Higher proportions of girls than boys achieve 5 or more passes at these levels (49 per cent for girls, 40 per cent for boys)[40]. Examination results of pupils attending special schools are significantly worse than for pupils in "mainstream" schools[103].

Evidence

Cohort studies show that those with low levels of educational achievement have poor adult health[104,105]. There are a number of interpretations of this relationship, which are not mutually exclusive. Level of education may act as a marker for other influences such as socioeconomic status, occupational level or lifestyle[106]. Educational attainment may be the route through which there are differential opportunities for income and employment, with their consequences on health[107]. Education may have a direct influence on health related behaviour: children who do well in education tend to report healthier behaviour in adult life in relation to diet, smoking and exercise[108]. In summary, although the extent to which education has an independent effect on health status, and the mechanisms by which it does so are not fully understood, it does appear to have an important influence. This influence may be seen as both potentiating, providing the trigger for healthier lifestyles and behaviour, and protective, providing access to employment opportunities and life chances that can protect individuals from disadvantage later in life.

However, those living in disadvantaged circumstances, who are most in need of the benefits of education, may be least able to gain access to them. Analyses suggest that inequalities in resource allocation to schools and provision for the renewal of school buildings have widened over the last two decades[109]. Schools in disadvantaged areas are more likely to be restricted in space and have the environment degraded by litter, graffiti, and acts of vandalism. This contributes to more stressful working conditions for staff and pupils. Children coming to school hungry or stressed as a result of their social and economic environment will be unable to take full advantage of learning opportunities. And stress, depression and social exclusion may reduce parents' capacity to participate in their children's education.

Whilst we recognise the constraints on what education can achieve due to unfavourable influences outside school, we are convinced that the education sector has important opportunities within its grasp to reduce inequalities in health. Furthermore, recent research has shown that there is marked variation in the effectiveness of secondary schools, as measured by educational attainment, even when measures of disadvantage amongst pupils have been taken into account[110]. Logic and equity argue that children most in need should receive increased resources for their education. Arrangements already exist through the Revenue Support Grant Formula to take account of deprivation. We consider that the effectiveness of the current resource allocation mechanisms should be reviewed and the distribution of educational resources should be more finely calibrated to the levels of disadvantage in the school.

Benefit

Enhanced education is likely to lead to health gains both directly, for instance through the adoption of health promoting behaviours and indirectly, for instance through a greater likelihood of employment.

4. We RECOMMEND the provision of additional resources for schools serving children from less well off groups to enhance their educational achievement. The Revenue Support Grant formula and other funding mechanisms should be more strongly weighted to reflect need and socioeconomic disadvantage.

Developing pre-school education

Out-of-home day care and pre-school education are two services which overlap in providing learning and care for those below current statutory school age. There is no clear and logical dividing line between them, as both must secure and promote children's healthy physical, emotional and intellectual development. The evidence which supports the effectiveness of out-of-home day care and pre-school education in promoting children's health and development also overlaps. It is presented in full here and summarised at recommendation 21.1 (on day care).

Inequality

Currently the provision of out-of-home day care and pre-school education services varies by area. Often the services are only available for those who can pay the full or subsidised fees[111]. A 1990 survey carried out by the Department of Health found that over 40 per cent of mothers of three and four year olds not attending day nursery would like their children to do so[112].

Evidence

Assessment of the most rigorous evaluations is found in a systematic review of randomised controlled trials of non-parental out-of-home day care before the age of 5 years[113]. This assessed 8 trials, all conducted in the USA. In total over two thousand children were randomly allocated to a group who received day care or to a group who did not. In 4 studies the day care started when the children were infants. Length of follow up ranged from 6 months to 27 years. Most of the studies targeted families of lower socioeconomic status, and nearly all included an element of home visiting and targeted parental training. The formal educational component varied, although all were concerned with the attainment of cognitive concepts. The review was not able to determine the effects of different parts of the programmes.

Although all studies showed that IQ was increased by participation in day care, this effect did not persist much after the end of this care. However, measures of educational performance tended to be persistently higher in the groups who received day care. Furthermore, there were no adverse effects of day care on behaviour. Other advantages included better educational, employment and financial achievement amongst mothers whose children received day care shown in some but not all of the studies. In one of the studies, the Perry Project (later called Highscope), follow up to 27 years of age showed that the people from the day care group were more likely to have advantageous social outcomes such as high school graduation, employment, fewer arrests, higher earnings, fewer teenage pregnancies and owning their own home. Furthermore, investment in pre-school provision in this project was associated with financial gain to society in the long term. Few outcomes measured health directly. Although the results of observational studies or cross-country comparisons have not always been consistent with those from experimental trials, weaknesses in design and evaluation have led to some of the apparently contradictory findings[111].

Overall the evidence suggests that pre-school education or day care may be especially effective in improving the achievement and health of the most disadvantaged children, although this will not necessarily bring them up to the level of their more advantaged contemporaries. The content and quality of the programmes are crucial. Social and emotional, as well as cognitive, objectives should be included, and high quality, including in the educator's own training, must be assured. Pre-school education may be a particularly good opportunity to involve parents in their children's education and to develop their own, particularly in enhancing parenting skills[114,115].

Benefit

Greater provision of high quality out-of-home day care and pre-school education should increase choice to use these services. Benefits include improved educational and social achievement in the children and perhaps for parents.

5. *We RECOMMEND the further development of high quality pre-school education so that it meets, in particular, the needs of disadvantaged families. We also recommend that the benefits of pre-school education to disadvantaged families are evaluated and,*

if necessary, additional resources are made available to support further development
(see also recommendation 21.1).

Developing health promoting schools

In the next two sections, we focus more specifically on the role of the education sector in protecting and promoting the current health of children and preparing them for life. We adopt a concept of the health promoting school in line with that of the World Health Organisation/Commission of the European Communities and Council of Europe initiative:

> "The health promoting school aims at achieving healthy lifestyles for the total school population by developing supporting environments conducive to the promotion of health. It offers opportunities for, and requires commitments to, the provision of a safe and health-enhancing environment"[101].

The three main components encompass:
- enhanced education for health through the formal curriculum,
- improvements in the physical and social environment for pupils and staff to work in, including paying attention to how the organisation of the school encourages or inhibits healthy living,
- expansion of school/wider community links[99].

Inequality

As already outlined, schools in more disadvantaged areas are more likely to have a poor physical environment for both pupils and staff and resource allocation may not be matched adequately to their greater need. The capacity of schools to provide a supportive environment for children, particularly those experiencing disadvantage, has been eroded over the past 15 years, through such measures as the deregulation of school meals of a minimum standard and subsidised price, reduction of entitlement to free school meals[116] and the reduction of access to playing fields, as school land has been sold off for housing development[109].

Cigarette smoking by school-aged children may be used as an indicator of health-promoting behaviour, although it is imperfect for this purpose. There is little social class gradient in the proportion of children who have ever smoked, although the average consumption of cigarettes is higher in lower socioeconomic groups[117]. However cigarette smoking in adolescence may be a marker of socioeconomic trajectory i.e. of where young people are going (class of destination) rather than where they have come from (class of origin)[118]. Thus there is a strong link between educational disadvantage and smoking status, with those leaving school at the minimum statutory age and without qualifications having higher rates of smoking in adolescence and early adulthood than their educationally advantaged peers. The association remains after parental socioeconomic status and parental smoking status are taken into account[118,119]. Drinking alcohol over the adult safe limit is reported more often by children in lower socioeconomic groups, although they are actually less likely to be regular or occasional drinkers than those in higher socioeconomic groups[117].

Evidence

With the important exception of children who are excluded or who truant, schools are one of the few contexts in which health promotion interventions can reach most children and young people.

A recent evaluation of health promoting schools found that this approach to health promotion can lead to gains in pupils' knowledge, attitudes, self-esteem and health behaviours, particularly in primary schools[120]. However, there is no evidence yet that these approaches differentially improve health in disadvantaged pupils or are particularly effective in disadvantaged areas.

Reviews of health promotion have tended to be topic-based. Although this approach is limited, the evidence of such reviews may be used to illustrate more general principles for implementation. Three examples are considered here. They are the promotion of life management skills, the prevention of substance misuse, and sex education.

The promotion of life management skills: emotional development and mental health may be enhanced by programmes which aim to increase competence in various areas, including problem-solving, communication, decision-making, and coping with emotions. An example is the "Life Skills" approach promoted by the World Health Organisation[121]. Such programmes have been associated with improved behaviour and social relationships[122,123]. Despite the importance of parenting in protecting and enhancing the health of families, many young people leave school without acquiring the knowledge and skills which enable them to plan and achieve becoming a successful parent. Parenthood education should be started at school and be based on the values of caring for children and the importance of relationships[124]. For life management skills in general, interventions with a number of components and within the context of a well-run and supportive school are more effective than single interventions[125,126].

Substance misuse: a recent review of interventions to prevent substance misuse among young people found that there were few rigorously evaluated interventions. However, the evidence reviewed did permit some broad conclusions which are relevant to school based health promotion programmes. These conclusions were, firstly, that programmes should recognise the specific needs of individuals and groups of individuals, and the differing social and cultural contexts in which substance misuse is engendered, initiated and maintained. Secondly, programme intensity should be high, 15 hours or more, with "booster" sessions to reinforce gains. Thirdly, the content of the programmes should include normative education which seeks to reduce perceptions of prevalence and acceptability of use. Fourthly, programmes should have a mix of elements which could include social influence and skills training. Of relevance to the approach of health promoting schools, the review found that programmes needed to have consistency of approach and context[127]. In addition, early programmes, delivered in primary schools, may be successful in the prevention of substance misuse[128].

Sex education: Features associated with successful education programmes include: timing, which should precede the onset of sexual activity; a combined approach to education and information about the provision of contraception; integration with psychological approaches and with other life management skills; context, emphasising responsible and caring relationships and a recognition of social influences and pressures; a focus on specific aims, such as delayed intercourse and safe intercourse; and the tailoring of the programmes to the needs of the group they are intended to serve[129,130].

These examples illustrate some principles of successful health promotion in schools. These include: early education; taking account of wider influences on health–related behaviour; and a supportive school setting. Some of these principles of successful interventions could be achieved by strengthening Personal, Health and Social Education (PHSE) within primary and secondary schools. In particular, the need for sex education to start before the onset of sexual activity indicates that it needs to start in primary schools.

Benefit

Successful health promotion at school should increase "life skills" with resultant improvements in many aspects of physical, mental and social health. Health promoting schools could also provide a supportive environment and be a context for building social cohesion and for community development. For health promotion in school settings to decrease inequalities in health, there must be attention to the particular needs of children experiencing disadvantage. Children who are excluded, or exclude themselves, from school are at high risk of adverse health outcomes and may be least able to benefit from school-based health promotion interventions.

6. We RECOMMEND the further development of "health promoting schools", initially focused on, but not limited to, disadvantaged communities.

Improving nutrition at school

Inequality

Compared with those from non-manual backgrounds, the diet of children aged $1\frac{1}{2}$ to $4\frac{1}{2}$ years from manual backgrounds has less emphasis on fruit juice, fruit and fresh vegetables (especially vegetables) and whole grain cereals and more emphasis on sweet foods and confectionery[131]. Comparable recent data are not available for school aged children.

Evidence

Children in families on Income Support or on income-based Job Seekers Allowance are entitled to free school lunch. About 15 per cent of pupils in England receive a free lunch and about a further 27 per cent pay for it[132]. School lunch is thus an important component of the diet of children from disadvantaged families. For this reason, and for nutrition education purposes, school lunches should reach reasonable nutritional standards. These should attempt to redress inequalities in the diet, such as fruit and vegetable consumption[131]. There is evidence that some members of poorer families go without food because of lack of money, although this is much more likely to be mothers than children[93,94]. The characteristics and extent of those at risk of such "food poverty" have not been fully determined. When they are, there may be a case for extending provision of free school lunches to include children from poor families who are not currently entitled, in order to relieve overall pressure on the family food budget, and improve the nutrition of other family members. Breakfast clubs are another promising innovation, but they have not been systematically introduced or evaluated. They may be linked with out of school activities and day care as well as being a vehicle for improving nutrition in deprived areas. Their use for the latter purpose needs to be evaluated.

Nutrition education is not only about the nutritional value of food, but about budgeting for food, and choosing, preparing and cooking it. These elements should be included in the curriculum. Nutrition provided at school and nutrition education are likely to be enhanced if there is a school food policy set in the context of a health promoting school[99,101,120]. Such a policy might, for instance, support the provision of healthy eating choices by avoiding the use of confectionery vending machines. The provision of free school fruit to reduce socioeconomic inequalities in fruit consumption has not been evaluated. Successful schemes may rely as much on the restriction of alternatives as on the provision of fruit *per se*[133]. The practicality of widespread application of such schemes is also unknown. School fruit might have as much a role in forming attitudes to future fruit consumption as in present consumption.

Benefit

Improvements in the nutrition of school-children should result in decreased levels of obesity and nutritional deficiencies, and in healthier eating patterns in adult life. In turn, this may decrease the risk of some chronic degenerative and other diseases of adult life, without increasing the risk of other conditions.

7. We RECOMMEND further measures to improve the nutrition provided at school, including: the promotion of school food policies; the development of budgeting and cooking skills; the preservation of free school meals entitlement; the provision of free school fruit, and the restriction of less healthy food.

3. Employment

Employment plays a fundamental role in our society. People are often defined, and define themselves, through what they do for a living. Sociological studies emphasise that not only is employment a primary source of status in industrialised countries like Britain, but it is also significant in providing purpose, income, social support, structure to life and a means of participating in society[134]. It has been called "the glue that keeps our society together"[135]. In such a context unemployment and stressful or hazardous working environments are potentially major risks to health for the population of working age and their families.

There are four main policy areas to address employment and health issues, which form the basis for our recommendations:

- ameliorating the health damage among people who experience unemployment, through ensuring adequate income levels for unemployed people and their families, for example; and matching services to the greater need related to unemployment;
- increasing training and education opportunities for population groups at greatest risk, to help prevent unemployment in the future;
- removing barriers to employment through, for example, the provision of adequate child care, family-friendly employment policies and employment generation;
- improving the employment conditions and health-enhancing quality of the work environment for people in employment.

Reducing unemployment and its effects on health

Inequality

By the International Labour Office (ILO) definition, two million people were unemployed in the UK in 1997, about 7 per cent of the economically active population of working age. Around half of all unemployed men and just under a third of unemployed women had been unemployed for one year or more[40]. The risk of being unemployed is much higher for young adults, people from minority ethnic groups, disabled people and for people in less skilled occupations and with fewer qualifications[40,45]. For example, unemployment rates are four times higher among unskilled workers than among professional groups[44], and three times higher for disabled than non-disabled people[136]. In addition to those recorded officially as unemployed, there are nearly 8 million people of working age in the UK who are classed as economically inactive because of long term sickness, for instance, or because they are looking after a family or have become discouraged in their search for work. A third of these report that they would like a job[40]. Many of the jobless households contain children, who share the consequences and living standards of their parents not being in employment. For example, of a total of 13.3 million dependent children in the UK in 1994–95, 4.1 million lived in households with no full-time worker, three quarters of whom were living in poverty (in a household below half of average income, after housing costs)[72].

Evidence

For a small minority, unemployment appears to lead to an improvement in health. But for the majority it tends to have a significant adverse effect on both physical and mental health. Unemployment is an important determinant of inequalities in the health of adults of working age in Britain, with people lower down the social scale being hardest hit[137–139]. Unemployed people are found to have lower levels of psychological well-being, ranging from symptoms of depression and anxiety to self-harm and suicide[140,141]. In relation to physical health, unemployment carries a higher risk of morbidity and premature mortality. In the latest analysis from the Longitudinal Study covering England and Wales, for example, mortality from all major causes was consistently higher than average among unemployed men. Among younger men, mortality from injuries and poisoning, including suicide, was particularly high. Unemployed women had high mortality from coronary heart disease and injuries and poisonings, including suicide[142]. The wives of unemployed men have been found to have an excess risk of death[143]. Even after taking account of the more disadvantaged circumstances of unemployed people, an excess risk of death of more than 20 per cent remains[142].

Explanations for how unemployment leads to poorer health centre on four main mechanisms: through increased poverty and hardship; through social exclusion (isolation, stigma); through changing health related behaviour; and through disrupting future work careers (people who experience a spell of unemployment are at greater risk of becoming unemployed again within the next two years)[144]. In relation to hardship, the financial consequences of unemployment are often instant and dramatic. Cohort studies of people entering unemployment show that, for many, their income was cut by half as they switched from wages to social security benefits[145,146]. The largest British cohort study in the 1980s showed that two thirds of unemployed people had a week's notice or even less, and only 1 in 10 received any form of redundancy payment. Two thirds were under 35, and most came from manual or lower service occupations, at the lower end of the pay scale and with low or no educational or technical qualifications[144]. Families with an unemployed head are at the highest risk of poverty[147]. Studies of the adequacy of state benefits identify unemployed households with dependent children as being particularly badly off[148–151].

Some of the excess morbidity and mortality associated with unemployment may be a result of people in poorer health being more likely to become unemployed, rather than vice versa. The evidence suggests that selection of unhealthy people into unemployment does indeed occur, but it is not the dominant factor explaining the observed relationship between unemployment and excess risk of ill-health. It does, however, illustrate the double disadvantage that people with chronic sickness or disability may face: their ill-health puts them at greater risk of unemployment, and the experience of unemployment in turn may damage their health still further.

Unemployment is associated with lower levels of educational attainment[152] and other skills. The lack of such skills may prove a barrier to obtaining employment[153] reinforcing earlier or other disadvantage. For example, Labour Force Survey Data indicate that 41 per cent of disabled people of working age have no educational qualifications, compared with 18 per cent of non-disabled people[154]. Unemployment is particularly high amongst young people. The rates of unemployment among people up to the age of 25 years are about twice as high as for all adult workers[155]. Schemes to raise levels of skills amongst people without a job, particularly young people, have been important components of Government policies over the last 20 years or so.

Evaluations of policies that have aimed to increase levels of skills among young people have reached differing conclusions. Some have concluded that such training increases likelihood of "a good job", whilst others have found that such success is very limited[156-160]. In particular, such schemes may fail the most disadvantaged by not addressing other problems, such as homelessness or lack of social support, which may present greater barriers to employment than lack of skills[161]. "Foyer" schemes are an example of a broader approach to disadvantage amongst unemployed young people. They consider the need for housing and social support as well as training and employment, but have yet to be thoroughly evaluated[162,163].

Many jobless households contain children, the majority living in poverty. Parents, especially lone parents, who wish to take up work may face several barriers. These include a lack of affordable child care, limited flexibility in parental leave and leave to care for sick children, and excessive and unsociable working hours. By comparison with many other member states of the European Union, the United Kingdom's policies in this area are limited. For instance, the UK has no provision for parental leave or leave to care for sick children, whereas half the (mainly European) 20 countries in a recent study had arrangements for leave to care for sick children[164]. The Inquiry welcomes the publication of the Government's white paper "Fairness at Work"[165], issued in May 1998, with its commitment to "family-friendly policies". We consider that this is an important, if modest, step in the right direction, and commend the further development of such policies. Consequently, with the exception of day care for children, we have not made a specific recommendation in this area.

But the removal of barriers to work for parents with dependent children, and higher levels of skills and additional training will achieve little unless there are jobs available. Indeed, lack of availability of employment may increase the sense of exclusion of people who are unable to gain employment despite adequate levels of skills[161]. It is outside the scope of the Inquiry to recommend specific policies on employment creation. However, we consider that increasing employment opportunities is crucial to reducing inequalities in health.

Benefit

Improved financial support during unemployment should improve material living conditions and resources needed for health, including access to food, heating, and shelter. It may also improve the ability of unemployed people to take part in the life of their communities – reducing social exclusion.

Policies aimed at the creation of employment opportunities, improved levels of education and training for young unemployed people, and removal of barriers to work for parents with dependent children should increase the chances of health enhancing employment in addition to other beneficial effects on health and its determinants, for example, income.

8. We RECOMMEND policies which improve the opportunities for work and which ameliorate the health consequences of unemployment. Specifically:

8.1 we recommend further steps to increase employment opportunities.

8.2 We recommend further investment in high quality training for young and long term unemployed people.

We recommend policies which will further reduce income inequalities, and improve the living standards of households in receipt of social security benefits (recommendation 3).

We recommend an integrated policy for the provision of affordable, high quality day care and pre-school education with extra resources for disadvantaged communities (recommendation 21.1).

Improving the quality of jobs

Inequality

For those in paid employment, there have been major changes in the nature of work over the past two decades. Along with greater labour market flexibility and deregulation of employment contracts has come greater job insecurity. Indeed, it could be considered that the concept of a secure "job for life" is now obsolete. While all sections of the workforce have been affected by these trends, less skilled manual workers at the lower end of the labour market have been affected the most, in terms of greater exposure to low paid, temporary and insecure employment[166–169].

There is also a growing recognition of the impact of stressful working conditions on health. Popular opinion tends to equate stress at work with pressure of work. Surveys which ask about self-perceived pressure of work have found that people in higher socioeconomic groups report such pressure more frequently[170]. However, evidence of health related harm is associated more with specific psychosocial factors such as imbalance between psychological demands and control, and lack of control at work[171]. Exposure to high demand and low control is more common among lower socioeconomic groups[172].

Evidence

A number of studies from the UK and elsewhere in Europe and from the USA show that an imbalance between psychological demands and control, and lack of control at work are associated with increased risk of coronary heart disease, musculoskeletal disorders, mental illness, and sickness absence[171–176]. As these psychosocial factors are related to the organisation of work, there are opportunities for change.

A recent review of international case studies on improving psychosocial health in the workplace found that it was possible to make improvements by tailoring changes to specific workplaces[177]. Examples included increasing the variety and understanding of the different tasks in a production process, workforce participation in identification of problems and their solutions, and altering shift patterns to make them less tiring and disruptive to workers' personal lives. Furthermore, some changes in workplace organisation resulted in improved productivity. Although effective changes were likely to be specific to particular workplaces, successful interventions had some common features[177]. They were: appropriate commitment and effort from management; support by management and the workforce; participation of the workforce in planning and implementation; and the creation of trust. Conversely, aspects which inhibited the success of policies included: schemes which directed attention away from difficult working conditions and attempted to treat the symptoms only; technical solutions alone, imposed from the top; and cases where management retained control over the dialogue.

Successful interventions follow principles of good management practice[178]. Current Health and Safety Executive (HSE) Guidance endorses this[179]. The enhancement of management skills in the current and future workforce is likely to bring about both a culture and practice which is amenable to health-promoting work organisation and practices. Good management practice may be engendered during school years, particularly in the acquisition of "life skills"[121] as a component of Personal, Health and Social Education, and within the context of health promoting schools. Enhancing the management skills of the current workforce, particularly in relation to the promotion of psychosocial health, may be aided by further guidance and development work by the HSE, such as extending the current "Good health is good business" campaign to include psychosocial health[180]. It has been suggested that good practice might also be encouraged by extending psychosocial health and safety issues to award schemes, such as "Investors in People". Other options include extending existing HSE regulations to encompass psychosocial health.

Evidence from Scandinavia suggests that good practice may also be promoted by explicit commitment and leadership from the national level[177,181]. In this respect, we welcome the Government's white paper "Fairness at Work", which has the stated aim of "putting a very minimum infrastructure of decency and fairness around people in the workplace"[165]. In pointing out that Britain now has the most lightly regulated labour market of any leading economy in the world, it explicitly acknowledges the unfairness of this situation – denying British citizens basic employment rights that are a matter of course elsewhere. Some of the measures proposed in the white paper have the potential to influence health related psychosocial conditions at work, in particular in relation to job security. Assessing the impact on health of existing and proposed employment policies, such as these and the Welfare to Work scheme, will be crucially important to inform future policy-making.

Benefit

Improved work practices, together with complementary employment policies, should decrease psychosocial ill health and its consequences, and may have other gains, including economic gains for the individual and society.

9. We RECOMMEND policies to improve the quality of jobs, and reduce psychosocial work hazards. Specifically;

9.1 *we recommend employers, unions and relevant agencies take further measures to improve health through good management practices which lead to an increased level of control, variety and appropriate use of skills in the workforce.*

9.2 *We recommend assessing the impact of employment policies on health and inequalities in health* (see also *recommendation 1*).

4. Housing and Environment

Shelter is a pre-requisite for health. However, people who are disadvantaged suffer both from a lack of housing and from poor quality housing. Furthermore, the fear of crime compounds the social exclusion of people living in disadvantaged areas. This section sets out inequalities in housing and the environment and health and summarises the evidence which we have concluded indicates areas for future policy development. These areas are improving the availability of housing, improving its quality and increasing the safety of the environment in which people live. The section also summarises the benefits which might result from such policies.

Improving the availability of housing

Inequality

As a result of housing policy in the 1980s and early 1990s, social rented housing – local authority and housing association homes – has increasingly become a housing sector for low income groups. People moving into social housing have tended to be families with children on the lowest incomes while those moving out have been older, with higher incomes and fewer children[182]. The result is an over-concentration and separation of households with high levels of need in areas with poor amenities.

The last 20 years have also seen a rapid increase in homelessness, with the numbers of officially homeless families peaking in the early 1990s[183]. In 1997, 165,690 households were estimated to be homeless. Of these 103,340 were officially homeless, that is they met the definition of homelessness laid down in the 1977 Housing (Homeless Persons) Act. The remainder were unofficially homeless, including rough sleepers – those without any accommodation at all – and hostel users[51]. Because it is difficult to be accepted as officially homeless without the presence (or imminent arrival) of children, the officially homeless population contains a large number of mothers and dependent children. Fifty seven per cent of officially homeless households had dependent children, and a further 10 per cent had a pregnant household member. Seven per cent had a household member vulnerable through mental illness[51]. Over a third of the officially homeless are drawn from minority ethnic groups[184]. By contrast, minority ethnic groups are not over-represented among the unofficial homeless population, which is older and predominantly male (70 per cent of hostel users and 85 per cent of rough sleepers are men)[184]. Young people constitute a significant and high risk sub-group among the unofficially homeless population[185].

Rough sleepers are also drawn disproportionately from those who have been in an institution such as prison or mental hospital or have been in local authority care.

Evidence

Very high mortality rates have been recorded for homeless people, particularly for rough sleepers and hostel users[186]. Surveys also point to high levels of health need among the homeless population. Forty five per cent of the bed and breakfast population have been found to experience psychological distress, compared to 20 per cent of the general population[184]. Rates of self-reported depression and anxiety are three times higher among those in bed and breakfast accommodation and ten times higher in rough sleepers. There is also an elevated prevalence of major mental disorders, most notably schizophrenia[184], and, among young homeless people, a high rate of attempted suicide[187].

In addition to their higher risk of mental health problems, people who are single and homeless have a higher prevalence of bronchitis, tuberculosis, arthritis, skin diseases, infections, problems related to alcohol and substance misuse, and higher rates of hospital admission[188-190]. People living in temporary accommodation of the bed and breakfast kind have high rates of some infections and skin conditions and children have high rates of accidents[191-195]. Living in such conditions engenders stress in the parents and impairs normal child development through lack of space for safe play and exploration[192]. Whilst cause and effect are hard to determine, at the very least homelessness prevents the resolution of associated health problems. For example: many young people recently made homeless do not have adequate access to health care[191]; and homeless people who are heavy drinkers may have less access to health services for all their needs, including treatment of health problems related to alcohol and substance misuse[196-199].

Availability of housing is related both to the quantity and quality of housing. The quality of the housing stock in Britain has steadily improved over this century but has been relatively stable since 1991. An estimated 1.5 million (7.5 per cent) homes are "unfit", a similar number to that in 1991[50]. Estimates of the additional social, rental or "affordable" housing required varies according to the factors taken into account when making predictions. For England, typical figures have been for 90,000 to 100,000 homes per year, although some estimates are lower. However, most research indicates a considerable deficit in such housing production at present[200,201]. Taken together with the plateau in the number of homes which are unfit, it is likely that present housing conditions will not improve over the next five years, and may worsen.

Neighbourhoods and the development of new residential areas may benefit from the principle of planning to promote a mix of housing tenures, employment status, household composition and age groups. This may avoid the problems of concentration and isolation of those suffering the greatest disadvantages[182,202-205], and the consequent overload on services.

Benefit

Although improvements in quantity and quality of housing are not certain to improve health, it is logical that they should do so. Such benefits would be on a range of health outcomes. Reducing official and unofficial homelessness would meet a basic health need of groups already vulnerable to poverty and ill-health, including families and mentally ill young people. If improvements are made through community-led development, this may also enhance social networks, with other potential benefits to health[206,207].

10. We RECOMMEND policies which improve the availability of social housing for the less well off within a framework of environmental improvement, planning and design which takes into account social networks, and access to goods and services.

11. We RECOMMEND policies which improve housing provision and access to health care for both officially and unofficially homeless people.

Improving the quality of housing

Inequality

Properties in bad condition are occupied disproportionately by single older people[208]. Minority ethnic groups are generally more likely to be living in poor housing than the white majority[209].

Forty per cent of all fatal accidents happen in the home[208]. Almost half of all accidents to children are associated with architectural features in and around the home[210]. Households in disadvantaged circumstances are likely to be the worst affected by such accidents[194]. Those living in high rise buildings, frequently those in lower socioeconomic groups, are more prone to serious accidents, such as falls[208]. Families living in temporary accommodation are also likely to suffer accidents in the home[195].

Evidence

Poor quality housing is associated with poor health[211,212]. Dampness is associated with increased prevalence of allergic and inflammatory lung diseases, such as asthma, independent of smoking and socioeconomic factors[212–214]. Unmodernised older properties have far higher heating costs than improved and modern homes[208].
A survey of older people in 1988 found that 25 per cent were using less heat than they wished, because of the cost[97]. Cold housing leads directly to hypothermia and may contribute to the excess of winter deaths seen in older people[208,215]. It also leads to "fuel poverty"[96]. Whilst the hazards of such poverty could be addressed by increasing the financial resources available to older people and others living on state benefits, a more direct approach would be to improve the energy efficiency, insulation and heating systems of affected housing. Mechanisms to do this include further development of building regulations for new and existing buildings and through

further development of Government schemes which subsidise improvements in existing properties. Current Government schemes, for example, the Home Energy Efficiency Scheme, may not reach homes most in need, such as the private rented sector.

Temporary accommodation tends to be ill-designed, ill-equipped and ill-maintained. Poor housing design, for instance changes in floor levels at door thresholds, contributes to seemingly minor accidents in older people, which may have grave consequences[208]. Disabled people are under-represented amongst owner occupiers, and rely heavily on local authority housing, especially for accessible dwellings. The stock of accessible housing is insufficient to meet the needs of disabled people, particularly for those using wheelchairs[216–218].

Smoke alarms are effective in reducing deaths from fire[219]. The use of smoke alarms, mostly battery operated, has increased in recent years but those most at risk, e.g. living in temporary accommodation, are least likely to have an alarm where they live[50]. Options to promote the use of smoke alarms include placing a duty of care on landlords to install and maintain smoke alarms and including them in fitness standards for existing buildings. Removal of other accident hazards in the home might also be achieved by changes to regulations and fitness standards.

Benefit

Improvement in energy efficiency in homes is likely to improve the health of occupants, both directly and by releasing their financial resources for other uses. It also has wider benefits in conserving energy. Removal of hazards in homes is likely to lead directly to reduced death and injury from accidents. Improvements in home design might allow disabled and older people to be cared for at home, with improvements in their quality of life.

12. *We RECOMMEND policies which aim to improve the quality of housing. Specifically:*

12.1 *we recommend policies to improve insulation and heating systems in new and existing buildings in order to further reduce the prevalence of fuel poverty.*

12.2 *We recommend amending housing and licensing conditions and housing regulations on space and amenity to reduce accidents in the home, including measures to promote the installation of smoke detectors in existing homes.*

Reducing the fear of crime and violence

Inequality

Crime and fear of crime can affect profoundly the quality of people's lives. Just over half of the 4 million incidents of contact crime – wounding, robbery and common assault – counted by the British Crime Survey in 1995 involved injury to the victim, usually bruising and scratches. Serious physical injury is rare. But anger, shock, fear and a sense of invasion of privacy are felt by many victims[220].

Not everyone is at equal risk of becoming a victim of crime. Young men, as well as being the most common perpetrators of crime, are also the most likely victims of street crime, especially physical assaults. Older people, especially women, are more likely to be victims of theft from the person. Crime tends to be concentrated in areas of social deprivation. Other indicators, such as the incidence of vandalism, graffiti, nuisance and substance misuse, are associated with levels of crime and can thus be useful markers of people's experience of crime, much of which is never reported to the police[221]. People from minority ethnic groups are at a greater risk of violent crime and of racial harassment[66,222].

Fear of crime can also be a cause of mental distress and social exclusion. In particular, women and older people tend to worry more about becoming victims and this may prevent them from engaging in social activities. People's fear of being a victim of crime may be well in excess of the actual risks. The British Crime Survey found that 4 per cent of men, aged over 16 years, and 18 per cent of women felt very unsafe walking in the area near their home at night. These figures increased to 8 per cent for men and 31 per cent for women if only people over the age of 60 years were considered, and were considerably higher if lesser degrees of concern about safety were included. Furthermore, 1 per cent of men and 4 per cent of women felt very unsafe in their own homes if alone and at night[220].

People who suffer from poor health are more likely to be victims of crime than those in good health. However, this may be because of the association of disadvantage with both victimisation and poor health, rather than poor health causing victimisation[220].

Evidence

There is increasing evidence to suggest that society level factors, and poverty and income inequality in particular, may be important underlying causes of crime[223,224]. Studies have described how widening income inequalities in countries like Britain and the US have been accompanied by a greater spatial separation of rich and poor[202]. This has led to a search for mechanisms which might explain the observed relationship between income inequality and its associated residential concentrations of poverty and affluence, on the one hand, and crime on the other. One hypothesis is that income inequality is related to crime via a depletion in social cohesion, as measured by high levels of mutual distrust and low levels of reciprocity between people living in the same neighbourhood, region, or society[224–226].

Although the evidence is incomplete, the link between income inequality, social cohesion and crime has important policy implications. It suggests that crime prevention strategies which only target the perpetrators and victims of crime and the high crime areas in which both groups live, will not achieve a significant reduction in crime unless they are accompanied by measures to reduce income inequality and promote social cohesion[224,226].

The most effective approaches to crime prevention are likely to be those which are integrated with wider social and economic policies for reducing health inequalities. In particular, pre-school education has been shown to have a long term effect on the incidence of criminal behaviour in early adult life[113,115]. Similarly, measures that address the welfare needs of young people are likely to have an impact on the incidence of youth crime[227].

There are a number of other measures which can help to protect local communities from high rates of crime and help people feel more secure. These measures include modifying the physical environment in such a way that crime is less likely to occur – for example, street lighting, changing the design, layout and landscaping of buildings; providing better surveillance – for instance concierge schemes, use of CCTV cameras and security alarms; and involving local police in "community policing", where officers spend more time on the beat, are proactive in identifying problems, and form partnerships with local people, businesses and other agencies. In this way, the expertise, knowledge and resources of local communities are used in helping to define, target and resolve problems[228].

Benefit

It is beyond the scope of this Inquiry to recommend particular approaches to prevent or reduce crime. However, there appears to be good evidence that crime and fear of crime is felt disproportionately by disadvantaged groups and that "upstream" policies, such as pre-school education, can reduce criminal behaviour in adolescence. There is also a general consensus that crime can be prevented through targeted policing and by involving local communities which itself may promote social cohesion[228]. However the relative benefits of different measures, including social and economic regeneration programmes and greater provision of services for young people, are not known.

13. We RECOMMEND the development of policies to reduce the fear of crime and violence, and to create a safe environment for people to live in.

We recommend policies which will further reduce income inequalities, and improve the living standards of households in receipt of social security benefits (recommendation 3).

5. Mobility, Transport and Pollution

The primary function of transport is in enabling access to people, goods and services[229]. In so doing it also promotes health indirectly through the achievement and maintenance of social networks. Some forms of transport, such as cycling and walking, promote health directly by increased physical activity and reduction of obesity. Lack of transport may damage health by denying access to people, goods and services and by diverting resources from other necessities. Furthermore, transport may damage health directly, most notably by accidental injury and air pollution.

Improving public transport

Inequality

In the 1991 Census, those living in accommodation rented from a housing association or local authority were nearly four times as likely to have no access to a car as those living in owner occupied housing (68 per cent compared to 19 per cent) and over six times less likely to have access to two or more cars (5 per cent compared to 32 per cent)[52]. In rural areas having no access to a car was less common than in urban areas (15 per cent compared to 34 per cent), and having access to two or more cars was more common (42 per cent rural areas, 22 per cent in urban areas). People living in rural areas were somewhat more likely than those living in urban areas to travel to work by car (69 per cent and 60 per cent respectively) but much less likely to use public transport if they had no car (23 per cent in rural areas, 49 per cent in urban areas)[54].

Evidence

Lack of access to transport is experienced disproportionately by women, children, disabled people, people from minority ethnic groups, older people and people with low socioeconomic status, especially those living in remote rural areas. Examples of lack of access include: people living in council housing, where poor access to transport may limit work and training opportunities[230,231]; higher prices and a restricted range of goods available to people whose lack of access to transport denies them opportunities to shop in supermarkets[232]; limited access to health care facilities for people without a car living in rural areas[233]; and environmental barriers in access to transport experienced by people with physical disabilities[217].

Higher traffic volumes result in feelings of insecurity, especially amongst families with children, and older people[234], and are associated with lower levels of non-traffic street level activity, such as walking. This can result in a community with limited potential for building or maintaining social networks[235]. Disadvantaged urban areas tend to be characterised by high traffic volume, leading to increased levels of air and noise pollution and higher rates of road traffic accidents without the benefits of access to private transport[229].

The cost of rail and local bus fares has risen by nearly one third in real terms since 1980, whereas motoring costs have decreased by 5 per cent[236]. Thus the increased cost of commonly used modes of public transport has had the most impact on those with lowest incomes. Consequently, use of transport may have declined amongst the least well off. A dramatic demonstration of this occurred in South Yorkshire. Prior to bus de-regulation in April 1986, South Yorkshire had a comprehensive and cheap public transport system, with decreasing prices in real terms and increasing usage. After de-regulation, bus fares rose by 250 per cent. Unemployed people and those who had retired reduced their journeys more than those in work (62 per cent and 60 per cent respectively compared to 37 per cent), as did school children (by 48 per cent). Social support networks suffered as travel to undertake informal caring roles became more difficult. This resulted in increased requests for statutory support services, including home helps[237-239]. Low incomes may be particularly strained in rural areas, where the lack of public transport makes car ownership a necessity[240].

Further development of a high quality, healthy transport system for the public, which is integrated with other forms of transport, for instance walking and cycling, and is affordable to the user, is crucial to the reduction of inequalities in health. We consider that it is beyond the scope of the Inquiry to recommend the mechanisms which might be used to improve and develop such a public transport system. However, suggestions made to us include the decentralisation of funding and responsibility for local transport within an overall policy framework, and providing suitable powers for statutory partnerships to set and monitor standards of public transport.

Benefit

Improved public transport should lead to improved access to people and facilities fundamental to health, such as family and friends, shops, parks and leisure facilities, and health care. This in turn should lead to improvement in quality of life and health. If transport is made more affordable than at present, this would release resources which might be used for health promoting activities and goods. Increased use of public transport by the general population would have the result of decreasing air and noise pollution which is suffered disproportionately by people experiencing disadvantage. A decrease in the use of cars would lead to a reduction of accidents. This is likely, but not certain, to be accompanied by a reduction in inequalities in accident rates.

14. We RECOMMEND the further development of a high quality public transport system which is integrated with other forms of transport and is affordable to the user.

Encouraging walking and cycling

Inequality

Pedestrian injury death rates for children in social class V are five times higher than for those in social class I[241], and are higher for boys than girls[25].

Evidence

The most health promoting and equitable forms of transport, walking and cycling, are vulnerable to the disadvantages imposed by motor vehicles[229]. There has been a post-war decline in walking and cycling, which has come about partly because of a sense of increased danger consequent on the rise in motor vehicle traffic volume[236]. There is also evidence of a high level of suppressed demand for cycling. Some disadvantaged groups, for instance children from families without a car, are more likely to make journeys by foot, cross more roads than those who have access to a car, and consequently are exposed to higher risks of a pedestrian accident[242].

Re-allocation of road space to provide more infra-structure for pedestrian and cycle route networks has been effective in increasing the use of these modes and decreasing accidents in some cities such as York. Other examples have been found in Europe[243]. Smaller schemes, such as Safe Routes to School, may also be effective[244]. Such schemes need to be sensitive to local circumstances and involve the local community in decision making and implementation. This is an important feature of successful community accident prevention interventions, and indeed any community intervention[219,245].

Benefit

Those engaged in walking and cycling would gain from increased physical exercise and its health benefits. If overall levels of walking and cycling increased, at the expense of the use of motor vehicles, then it is likely that accident rates and levels of air pollution would fall. The burden of both falls disproportionately on people experiencing disadvantage.

15. We RECOMMEND *further measures to encourage walking and cycling as forms of transport and to ensure the safe separation of pedestrians and cyclists from motor vehicles.*

Reducing the use of motor vehicles

Inequality

The main cause of air pollution is emissions from motor vehicles, which include particulates and ozone[246]. About a third of households have no access to a car[42], and these tend to be households with lower income[52]. Yet air pollution is more common close to roads and road junctions, and in inner urban areas[247-249], places which are often characterised by other indicators of disadvantage[229]. Thus the burden of air pollution tends to fall on people experiencing disadvantage, who do not enjoy the benefits of the private motorised transport which causes the pollution.

Evidence

A recent report by the Department of Health's Committee on the Medical Effects of Air Pollutants (COMEAP) concluded that air pollution in urban areas, in the form of particulate matter, is responsible for bringing forward 8,100 deaths a year and bringing forward or creating an additional 10,500 hospital admissions for respiratory disease a year. In addition, in both urban and rural areas in the summer months, ozone is responsible for bringing forward 12,500 deaths and bringing forward or creating an additional 9,900 hospital admissions for respiratory disease per year. COMEAP also confirmed their previously stated view that the association between air pollution and mortality and morbidity is causal[250].

Two options to reduce air pollution associated with motor vehicles are to decrease their use and to decrease their capacity to pollute[246]. The latter is likely to be a lesser effect, and any success in reducing emissions of pollutants will be outweighed if the use of and number of motor vehicles continues to increase. The annual increase in the amount of road traffic from 1993 to 1995 was over 2 per cent. Apart from isolated periods road traffic volume has increased steadily since the 1950s. Projections estimate that road traffic will increase between 55 per cent and 87 per cent between 1995 and 2025 (figure 15). Most of this increase will be cars[246,251].

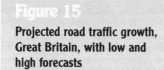

Projected road traffic growth, Great Britain, with low and high forecasts

Source:
Royal Commission on Environmental Pollution (1997)[246]

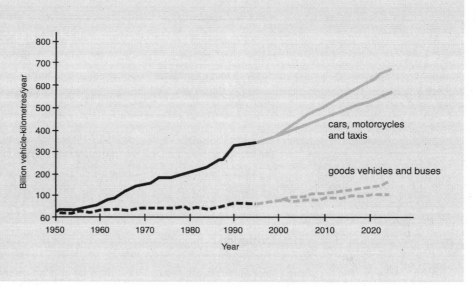

Reduction of the use of motor cars appears to depend on the availability and acceptability of alternative modes of transport. These include walking, cycling and public transport. Walking and cycling may be particularly important in reducing air pollution as they could replace short car journeys under "cold-start" conditions, which cause a disproportionate amount of pollution[246]. Car journeys to school are a typical example. In order to be able to compete with the attractions of travel by car, an effective public transport system must be integrated: that is it must be a system in which people can change quickly and easily from one route to another and from one mode of transport to another. It must also be a financially attractive option, which may mean subsidising the service for all users, not just for those from disadvantaged groups.

Benefit

Reduction of the use of motor vehicles would decrease air pollution and probably also reduce road traffic accidents. The benefit of these decreases is likely to be gained most by people experiencing disadvantage, who currently bear much of the burden. Use of alternative modes of transport might also reduce inequalities in health through the benefits that a more effective public transport system would bring to those without access to private transport. Increased opportunities for walking and cycling should increase overall health, but the effect on inequalities in health is unknown and would depend on how different sections of the population took up these opportunities.

16. We RECOMMEND *further steps to reduce the usage of motor vehicles to cut the mortality and morbidity associated with motor vehicle emissions.*

Reducing traffic speed

Inequality

Motor vehicle traffic accidents are a major cause of preventable deaths, particularly in younger age groups. For children and for men aged 20–64 years, mortality rates for motor vehicle traffic accidents are higher in lower socioeconomic groups[29,241]. For instance, there would be 600 fewer deaths in men aged 20–64 years from motor vehicle traffic accidents each year if all men had the same death rates as those in social classes I and II combined[32]. For children and adults over 65 years mortality rates from such accidents are higher in those born on the Indian sub-continent. For adults aged 15–24 and over 65 years rates are higher for those born in Ireland[252]. There are also differences in standardised mortality rates from motor vehicle traffic accidents around the country. The standardised mortality rate in 1996 varied from 59 in London to 122 in the East Midlands[253]. Age standardised rates are three times higher for males than females[25].

Evidence

Speeding generally exacerbates risks for all road users, but particularly for pedestrians and cyclists. The chance of a pedestrian being seriously injured or killed if struck by a car is 85 per cent if the car is travelling at 40 mph, 45 per cent at 30 mph and 5 per cent at 20 mph[254]. Speeding is common, and speed limits are broken by most motorists in urban and rural areas, using all types of vehicle, whatever the time of day, day of week, or month of year[255].

Environmental modification of existing roads or design of new roads which has the effect of "traffic calming" reduces speed of traffic and, by effectively excluding heavy goods vehicles, also reduces noise pollution[256]. Further, it provides a better environment for play and other community based street-level activities[257]. Introduction of 20 mph zones is associated with, on average, a 61 per cent drop in pedestrian casualties and a 67 per cent drop in child pedestrian and cyclist casualties[254]. As speeding is common, stricter enforcement of current limits may also be effective. For example, the use of speed cameras typically brings a casualty reduction of around 28 per cent[254]. To reduce inequalities these measures might need to be introduced preferentially in disadvantaged areas.

Benefit

A reduction in the speed of motor vehicles should reduce the risks of serious injury or death from road traffic accidents. It may also enhance the environment for other activities such as play for children, and reduce pollution.

17. We RECOMMEND further measures to reduce traffic speed, by environmental design and modification of roads, lower speed limits in built up areas, and stricter enforcement of speed limits.

Making public transport affordable for pensioners and disadvantaged groups

Inequality

Lack of access to transport is experienced disproportionately by older people and people from low income groups, especially those living in rural areas[229,233].

Evidence

Older and disabled people are more likely to have low incomes and to be reliant on public transport. The price of public transport is thus a critical issue in their mobility. The well documented change in use of buses in South Yorkshire illustrates the degree to which older people's use of public transport is determined by price[238,239].

About 10.5 million older people are eligible for concessionary fares in Great Britain, in addition to people who are disabled, registered blind and those with impaired mobility. Concessionary fare schemes vary considerably in different parts of the country. In London, there is a statutory scheme enabling the issue of permits to older and disabled people for travel on local buses, London Underground and suburban rail. The permit is free and travel is free after the morning peak. Outside London, local authorities have discretion to decide which form of concession to offer. Options include free travel, free or purchased permits which then allow free or reduced fare travel, or fares reduced by fixed percentages. Some authorities, for instance within the West Midlands Metropolitan Area, offer similar schemes to the statutory scheme in London. A recent survey found that most authorities (97 per cent) operate a scheme, but the many different types offered means that the cost of transport to the user varies considerably from place to place. In some places concessions are quite limited[258]. Furthermore, uptake of concessions is lower in areas of low population density, and is only 39 per cent in rural areas[259].

Benefit

Subsidised travel for older and disabled people should reduce a current barrier to health promoting opportunities.

18. We RECOMMEND concessionary fares should be available to pensioners and disadvantaged groups throughout the country, and that local schemes should emulate high quality schemes, such as those of London and the West Midlands.

6. Nutrition and the Common Agricultural Policy

By an immense programme of subsidies to agricultural production, the Common Agricultural Policy (CAP) has helped ensure the security of Europe's food supply since the end of World War II. Although this in itself has made an important contribution to health, the gain must be balanced against the consequent increased cost of food to the consumer. The range of foods affected includes cereals, meat, eggs, dairy produce, sugar, fruit and vegetables. Although the scale of the premiums varies across this range according to market conditions, and is difficult to measure, it is often substantial.

The significance of the CAP to inequalities in health is that the subsidies have maintained food prices usually at a higher level than necessary. As the poor spend a higher percentage of their income on food than the better off, the result is that the higher prices have the greatest impact on those least able to bear them. This is borne out by the reappearance of food poverty – going without food because of lack of money – in various parts of Europe including Britain[116,261].

The impact of CAP on the health of the less well off

Unfortunately, although the health impact of some of the individual programmes have been evaluated, there is no comprehensive review of the CAP's impact on the food budgets of the less well off, and through this on inequalities in health. We believe that this should be given a priority. CAP is by far the largest budget within the European Union – around 40 billion ecu a year (£32.5 billion)[262] – and is currently being reviewed as part of the Agenda 2000 programme in preparation for the next round of the World Trade Organisation talks. However, we are concerned that the health and health inequalities aspects of the CAP should be recognised and form part of this wider debate. We see an opportunity for the UK Government to build on the success of its European Union Presidency by hosting a conference to debate the implications of CAP on health and health inequalities.

The CAP's focus has been on raw food production. Its structure has meant that subsidies have led to surpluses so that half the budget provides subsidies to storage or export. The juxtaposition of "butter and meat mountains" and rising food poverty led to unfavourable publicity and the creation of a Surplus Food Scheme designed to redistribute food to the less well off. This small but significant "social policy" outcome of the CAP tends to be limited only to storable goods such as dried or frozen foods rather than fresh foods such as fruit and vegetables. The practical problems of redistribution have so far ruled out the use of fresh fruit and vegetables on the Surplus Food Scheme[263]. Even within this scheme, we believe that there is scope for more effective use of subsidies to reflect nutritional and public health goals, perhaps directed at school-aged children.

From the nutritional point of view, the situation with regard to the supply of fresh fruit and vegetables is currently the most unsatisfactory aspect of the CAP. At a time when data have pointed to the protective effects of fruit and green vegetables in the prevention of cancer and coronary heart disease[264,265], large sums of money are being spent in the destruction of these products. This amounted to 2.5 billion kilos of fruit and vegetables at a cost of 390 million ecu in 1993–94. Notwithstanding changes which have reduced the amount of compensation paid on such produce, it is our view that this policy needs to be reviewed, taking into account estimates of the "health gain" that would be derived from the supply of these foods at subsidised prices.

19. We RECOMMEND *a comprehensive review of the Common Agricultural Policy (CAP's) impact on health in general and inequalities in health.*

19.1 *We recommend strengthening the CAP Surplus Food Scheme to improve the nutritional position of the less well off.*

Increasing the availability and accessibility of food

Inequality

Food consumption varies between different socioeconomic groups. People in lower socioeconomic groups tend to eat less fruit and vegetables, and less food which is rich in dietary fibre. These patterns tend to hold true over all age groups in which they have been examined, from birth to 64 years. As a consequence, those in lower socioeconomic groups tend to have low intakes of anti-oxidant and other vitamins, and some minerals, especially relative to intakes in higher socioeconomic groups[35,55–58].

Even within low income groups, there are differences in nutrient intake which are related to income. The 20 per cent of Income Support claimants with compulsory deductions for rent or fuel have very restricted spending on food, and their resulting diets are far below reference values for intakes of iron, calcium, dietary fibre and vitamin C. This is even more likely if adults in the family smoke[94]. Furthermore, there is some evidence that such inequalities in nutrition, at least for some nutrients, have increased over the last 15 years[55].

There are also pronounced differences in diet by gender. Women are more likely than men to eat wholemeal bread, fruit and vegetables at least once per day and to drink semi-skimmed milk. They are less likely to drink alcohol heavily[35,53]. However, nutrient intakes of iron, calcium, magnesium, vitamin B12 and folate are lower in women than men, especially in women from lower socioeconomic groups. Many of the differences can be accounted for by the lower total food and energy intakes of women. An adequate intake of calcium appears to be an important component of bone health, reducing the risk of osteoporosis and fracture, although the evidence is incomplete[266–268]. Vulnerable groups, such as adolescent girls and older women, should therefore avoid low calcium intakes. The main dietary sources of calcium are milk, milk products and cereal products. Vitamin D is essential for calcium absorption and utilisation. Adequate dietary intake of vitamin D is necessary if skin synthesis is likely to be sub-optimal, for instance, for older people who are housebound or those who wear concealing clothing, and for vulnerable groups, such as pregnant and lactating women[269]. The best method of achieving adequate intake through supplementation of high risk groups is currently the subject of multi-centre trials.

Women may be more likely to under-report the quantity of their diet than men, and they are also more likely to diet. The relatively low intakes in women may partly reflect low intakes in a substantial proportion of women who are dieting at any single survey point[270]. The association between a mother's physique before and during pregnancy and cardiovascular risk in her children in later life suggests that her nutrition may have important long term effects on the health of the next generation[271-275]. The prevalence of dieting in women, especially young women, is a cause for concern.

Evidence

The evidence that links diet and nutrition to health and inequalities in health is, in the main, based on research showing that nutritional risk factors for disease and higher rates of nutrition related diseases cluster in disadvantaged groups. For example, dental caries are more prevalent in children in lower socioeconomic groups, and children in these groups have higher intakes of sweet drinks and snacks between meals – risk factors for caries. Death from stomach, oropharyngeal and oesophageal cancer is more common in lower socioeconomic groups and has been linked to low intake of fruit and vegetables, also more common in lower socioeconomic groups. Cerebrovascular disease is more common in lower socioeconomic groups and is associated, possibly through the intermediate risk factor of hypertension, with consumption of salty, energy dense foods which are high in sodium and low in magnesium and with low consumption of fruit and vegetables. This pattern of diet is more common in lower socioeconomic groups[276].

However, the effect of policies aimed at changing nutrition or single nutrients in the diet may be difficult to predict, given the sometimes complex link between diet, nutritional status and health. Thus our recommendations are based on enabling those who are disadvantaged to have the choice to purchase and consume a balanced diet[269].

Benefit

Reductions in inequalities in nutrition should lead to reductions in diseases which have nutrition-related risk factors. These include some types of cancer, cardiovascular disease, osteoporosis, anaemia, dental disease, and obesity and hypertension, and their complications. The extent to which these will be preferentially reduced in particular groups, for instance those from lower socioeconomic groups, is unpredictable. For instance, a reduction in total fat intake is a current recommendation to the whole population, based on the premise that this will lead to a reduction in average plasma cholesterol levels, which in turn will lead to reduced coronary heart disease. As, for a given level of plasma cholesterol, people from lower social classes have higher rates of coronary heart disease than those from higher social classes, an overall reduction in average plasma cholesterol may have a greater effect in reducing coronary heart disease in lower social classes[277].

20. We RECOMMEND policies which will increase the availability and accessibility of foodstuffs to supply an adequate and affordable diet.

Reducing food poverty and improving retail provision

Inequality

Households in the bottom tenth of the income distribution spend an average of 29 per cent of their disposable income on food (after allowance for housing costs) compared to 18 per cent for those in the top tenth[278]. People in low socioeconomic groups buy more efficiently than high income households, obtaining more grams of food of any type per pound spent. However, they also spend more on foods richer in energy and high in fat and sugar, which are cheaper per unit of energy than foods rich in protective nutrients, such as fruit and vegetables[116]. It also costs them more to shop because the physical inaccessibility of large retail food outlets necessitates expenditure on transport or the higher prices in small local shops[232]. The food budget is susceptible to "squeezing" to meet other demands, partly because it is a large proportion of low income households' budgets and partly because it is not protected. Rent and other deductions may be made compulsorily which places additional strain on the remainder of the budget[94].

Food poverty is experienced by some people in low income groups, particularly single mothers[93-95,116]. The diets of families living on low income may also lack choice and variety, a consequence of the expense of supplying choice and the associated potential for waste of food[93,279,280].

Evidence

Economies of scale allow food sold in supermarkets to be cheaper and to cover a wider range than that in smaller "high street" stores[232]. Furthermore, there is a paradox in that a "healthy" basket of food has been found to cost more in disadvantaged areas than in affluent areas[232,281]. The increasing tendency to out of town supermarkets has led to the creation of "food deserts" where cheap and varied food is only accessible to those who have private transport or are able to pay the costs of public transport, if this is available. People on low income, and in particular women and older people, are less likely to be able to drive or have access to a car, and price is a significant determinant of their ability to utilise public transport[40,282]. The cost of transport may add a considerable amount to the cost of food shopping[283,284]. Thus access to a cheaper and wider range of food is most restricted for some of the groups who need it most.

Currently, planning authorities do not have to consider the impact on low income groups when considering the development of retail food outlets. However, some local authorities have addressed the accessibility of food retail provision in disadvantaged areas, for instance by rate concessions to encourage retailers in these areas.

Town and country planning policies could be amended or emphasised to ensure that development of retail food outlets do not have an adverse effect on those most vulnerable to poor nutrition[285].

Benefit

People on low incomes eat less healthily partly because of cost, rather than lack of concern or information[286,287]. Therefore increased availability of affordable "healthy" food should lead to improved nutrition in the least well off.

20.1 *We recommend the further development of policies which will ensure adequate retail provision of food to those who are disadvantaged.*

We recommend policies which will further reduce income inequalities, and improve the living standards of households in receipt of social security benefits (recommendation 3).

We recommend the further development of a high quality public transport system which is integrated with other forms of transport and is affordable to the user (recommendation 14).

Reducing sodium in processed foods

Inequality

The best measure of salt in the diet is 24 hour urinary sodium excretion. There are scant data on the social distribution of this in Britain. The INTERSALT study showed that people of lower education, world-wide, had higher levels of sodium excretion. This was confirmed for the UK INTERSALT centres. This, together with higher rates of obesity and lower intakes of foods rich in potassium, places those from lower socioeconomic groups at higher risk of hypertension and its related risks. Average blood pressure increases as social class decreases, i.e. it is higher in lower social classes, although the gradient is not pronounced, especially in men[37]. However, at any level of blood pressure people from lower socioeconomic groups appear to be more vulnerable to the associated diseases, as evidenced by their higher rates of coronary heart disease and stroke[29].

Evidence

Less than 20% of sodium intake is discretionary and added in cooking or at the table. Most of the rest is in processed food[264]. Lower income groups have higher consumption of processed foods rich in sodium, for instance white bread, meat products (such as pies) and processed vegetables, other than frozen[55]. Observational studies, trials and animal studies all point to a relation between sodium intake and blood pressure. A review of this evidence led the Department of Health's Committee on Medical Aspects of Food Policy to recommend a one third reduction in sodium intake in the British diet[264], although other reviews have been more cautious[288]. A reduction in sodium intake, combined with a reduction in obesity and heavy drinking and an increase in potassium intake, would lower mean blood pressure in the population and hence reduce cardiovascular disease.

Benefit

Reduction of sodium in processed foods should reduce average blood pressure for the whole population. This may be of greater benefit in lower socioeconomic groups because of their increased susceptibility to the complications of hypertension, coronary heart disease and stroke.

20.2 We recommend policies which reduce the sodium content of processed foods, particularly bread and cereals, and which do not incur additional cost to the consumer.

7. Mothers, Children and Families

We recommend a high priority is given to policies aimed at improving health and reducing health inequalities in women of childbearing age, expectant mothers and young children (recommendation 2).

Reducing poverty in families

This section sets out inequalities in wealth in families, and summarises the evidence for areas of policy development and the benefits which may result from such policies. Our recommendations relate firstly to the removal of barriers to work, for parents who wish to combine work with parenting, by increasing access to day care. Secondly they relate to enabling those who wish to devote full-time to parenting to do so, by improving the living standards of households in receipt of social security benefits.

Inequality

The increased risk of poverty amongst families with young children has been documented in the text accompanying recommendation 3. Some parents find themselves in a benefit dependent poverty trap and would seek work if affordable child-care was available. However for parents in low income groups there is a shortage of affordable and appropriate child-care, both for pre-school and school-aged children[289-291]. A study of 20 countries, mostly European, found that the UK had the highest child-care costs of all countries, amounting to a quarter of average earnings[164]. At that time there were no public subsidies for child-care.

Evidence

Out-of-home day care and pre-school education are two services which overlap in providing learning and care for those below current statutory school age. There is no clear and logical dividing line between them, as both must secure and promote children's healthy physical, emotional and intellectual development. The evidence which supports the effectiveness of out-of-home day care and pre-school education in promoting children's development also overlaps. It is presented in the text supporting recommendation 5 (pre-school education) and is summarised here.

Evaluation of non-parental out-of-home day care before the age of 5 years has found that it is associated with improvement in a range of educational and social measures, some of which have been documented many years after the care. It is important to note that the best known studies are of the effect of centre-based day care, and it is not known whether the same advantages are found with care provided in other settings. All of the assessed studies contained educational components as part of the intervention programme, and nearly all an element of home visiting and/or parental training. It is not possible to assess which components of these multi-faceted programmes were effective. However it is clear that quality, including quality in training carers, is crucial: indeed poor quality care may be damaging[113,115]. There is no evidence for an optimal age for out-of-home day care[113,115]. The effect of early separation of parent and child on the child's social and emotional development and attachment remains a subject of controversy.

Benefit

Greater provision of high quality out-of-home day care, especially if integrated with pre-school education, should increase the availability of these services. Since it is easier to combine paid work and family responsibilities when parents have access to high quality day care, it is a potential mechanism to alleviate family poverty for parents who wish to combine work with parenting[292]. Other benefits include improved educational and social achievement in the children, and the potential for beneficial effects on the psychosocial health of parents and on their opportunities for education and training.

21. We RECOMMEND policies which reduce poverty in families with children by promoting the material support of parents; by removing barriers to work for parents who wish to combine work with parenting; and by enabling those who wish to devote full-time to parenting to do so. Specifically:

21.1 we recommend an integrated policy for the provision of affordable, high quality day care and pre-school education with extra resources for disadvantaged communities (see also: recommendation 5).

In making this recommendation, we commend the Government's commitment to a national Child-care Strategy as a first step in reducing inequalities in this area.

We recommend further reductions in poverty in women of childbearing age, expectant mothers, young children and older people should be made by increasing benefits in cash or in kind to them (recommendation 3.1).

We recommend measures to increase the uptake of benefits in entitled groups (recommendation 3.3).

Improving the health and nutrition of women and children

This section describes how inequalities in nutrition in women and children influence health. Our recommendations here are focused on improving the health and nutrition of women of childbearing age and their children, with priority given to the elimination of food poverty and the reduction of obesity.

Inequality

The babies of women in disadvantaged groups are more likely to have reduced growth rates in utero. Babies with fathers in social classes IV and V have a birthweight which is on average 130 grams lower than that of babies with fathers in social classes I and II[34]. Birthweight also varies by mothers country of birth. Babies whose mothers were born on the Indian sub-continent are on average 200 grams lighter than those of mothers born in the United Kingdom[34].

For women, obesity is more prevalent in lower social classes. There is a gradient of decreasing obesity with increasing social class. Twenty five per cent of women in social class V are obese compared to 14 per cent in social class I[37].

Evidence

Reduced growth in fetal life is associated with increased mortality and morbidity in the first year of life[293,294], and throughout childhood[295–297]. People who had low birthweight, or who are thin or stunted at birth, are at increased risk of cardiovascular disease and the disorders related to it in later life[21]. These associations cannot be explained by confounding variables operating in adult life. Reduced fetal growth is more common in deprived areas of Britain[298]. Birthweight is determined by the weight and height of the mother, which in turn reflects her own growth in childhood. The physique of mothers is also related to later disease in their children. Children of women who are thin, having either a low body mass index (weight/length^2) or thin skinfolds are at increased risk of developing non-insulin dependent diabetes and raised blood pressure in adult life[271–273].

The generally agreed 'healthy diet' in pregnancy may have long term benefits in reducing the baby's later risk of cardiovascular disease without greatly influencing birthweight[271,275]. Mothers reliant on state benefits may not be able to afford a healthy diet[83,95] and may go short of food in order to feed their children[93,94]. In the United States guaranteeing a minimum income to pregnant women has been shown to increase birthweight[91], although the mechanism is unknown.

Children of women who are overweight are also at increased risk of coronary heart disease as adults[274]. This effect is stronger among women with short stature. Short, overweight women are more common among low socioeconomic groups. Obesity is entrained during childhood and adolescence[299]. The rates of obesity in children are increasing, but there are no marked differences between social classes[300]. However, the effects of obesity on the development of coronary heart disease, non-insulin dependent diabetes and hypertension are more severe in people who had low birthweight[301-304].

Thus a baby's long term health is related to the nutrition and physique of its mother. Policies in this area should promote the avoidance of excessive thinness or obesity and a healthy diet for women of childbearing age. They should also promote avoidance of excessive weight gain in children.

Benefit

Improvement in the diet of girls and women is likely to bring improvements not only in their own health, but in the health of their children. Avoidance of obesity similarly benefits both the mother and her child. The effects of mothers' nutrition on their children's health will take more than one generation to alter. An approach which starts with both mothers and children is likely to bring the most rapid benefits.

22. We RECOMMEND policies which improve the health and nutrition of women of childbearing age and their children with priority given to the elimination of food poverty and the prevention and reduction of obesity. Specifically:

we recommend further reductions in poverty in women of childbearing age, expectant mothers, young children and older people should be made by increasing benefits in cash or in kind to them (recommendation 3.1).

We recommend further measures to improve the nutrition provided at school, including: the promotion of school food policies; the development of budgeting and cooking skills; the preservation of free school meals entitlement; the provision of free school fruit; and the restriction of less healthy food (recommendation 7).

We recommend a comprehensive review of Common Agricultural Policy's (CAP's) impact on health in general and inequalities in health (recommendation 19).

We recommend policies which will increase the availability and accessibility of foodstuffs to supply an adequate and affordable diet (recommendation 20).

Promoting breastfeeding

Inequality

Babies of fathers from social class I are more likely to be breastfed at birth than those from social class V, but this difference has decreased over the period from 1985–1995. Continued breastfeeding is much less common in lower social classes[59].

Evidence

Breastfeeding decreases the incidence and severity of many infections of infancy, and may protect from other infant and later adverse health outcomes. Breastfeeding may also protect the short and long term health of the mother[305].

Randomised controlled trials have shown that support to mothers during pregnancy, labour, and after birth increases not only initiation of breastfeeding, but also continuation and exclusivity, in other words breastfeeding only, without bottle feeding. Prenatal interventions tested include peer counsellors and education programmes tailored to women from specific cultural backgrounds. Continuous emotional support during labour provided by a trained – professional or lay – support person has been found to promote continued breastfeeding, as well as providing other benefits – for instance, reduced rates of Caesarean section[306]. Help with the practicalities of breastfeeding decreased early problems and increased duration of breastfeeding[307]. Some of these interventions were tested in particular disadvantaged groups (people living on low income)[308] and women from minority ethnic groups[309]. Evidence that they are differentially effective among people experiencing disadvantage is lacking.

Other measures of encouraging breastfeeding are based on increasing the acceptance and practicability of breastfeeding, especially outside the home. Such measures might include discussion of breastfeeding issues in Personal, Health and Social Education for school-children (see recommendation 6), using media advocacy and other publicity, and encouraging the provision of facilities for breastfeeding in shops and public places.

Benefit

Increased rates of breastfeeding should decrease the incidence of infant infection. The interventions suggested which do or could provide more support to the mother should also lead to other health gains in the mother and baby. It is unknown whether such interventions can be developed to be particularly effective in disadvantaged groups.

22.1 *We recommend policies which increase the prevalence of breastfeeding.*

Fluoridating the water

Inequality

Overall dental health in children is improving. The mean number of teeth with any known decay in children under 5 years has fallen over the last 10 years. However, the differential in the number of decayed teeth between those in classes IV and V and those in classes I, II and IIIN has increased, from an excess of 17 per cent in 1983 to one of 70 per cent in 1993[310,311]. The proportion of children who have an experience of dental decay also varies by area and by age. But at each age children living in the north have more dental decay than those living in the midlands and the south[312].

For example, at 5 years children living in the North West NHS Region show a 59 per cent excess compared with those in the South Thames NHS Region. At 12 years there is a 75 per cent excess[312].

Evidence

Fluoridation of the public water supply has been shown to reduce dental caries, especially amongst socially deprived communities in the UK and Australia[313,314]. Water fluoridation provides benefits for everyone but the effects are more pronounced in people in lower social classes[313,315], particularly in primary dentition. The Water Fluoridation Act (1985) and associated guidance from the Department of Health (HC/87/18) placed the responsibility for decisions about water fluoridation with health authorities. Following a request from a health authority, water undertakers may fluoridate the water supply. Although the Department of Health guidance indicates that the "chief concern" of water undertakers "will be the technical feasibility of water fluoridation", in practice water undertakers have interpreted the word "may" in the Act as giving them very wide discretion. Since the Water (Fluoridation) Act 1985 received Royal Assent (30 October 1985), no new fluoridation scheme has been introduced. (Those schemes implemented in the West Midlands had legally binding agreements before the Act.) To date, over 60 health authorities have completed the publicity and consultation required by the Act but cannot have their decisions on fluoridation implemented. Amendment of the Act would ensure fluoridation of the water supplies in areas where this has been recommended following the present legal processes.

Benefit

Fluoridation of water supplies should decrease inequalities in dental caries between areas, and between socioeconomic groups. Although benefit will at first be restricted to children, in time it will become evident in adults. The balance of scientific evidence is against harmful effects on health of fluoridation.

A relatively minor change is needed to the Act. As the process for public debate and decision-making would not be changed by the proposed amendment, arguments for and against fluoridation could continue to be considered as now.

22.2 *We recommend the fluoridation of the water supply.*

Reducing the prevalence of smoking in pregnancy

Inequality

Over the ten years from 1985 to 1995 there has been a slight decrease in the proportion of women smoking during or before pregnancy (39 to 35 per cent). Smoking prevalence during pregnancy is higher for manual than non-manual groups. Women from households in social class V are four times more likely to smoke in pregnancy than those in social class I[59].

Evidence

Maternal smoking is associated not only with reduced birthweight, but also with an increased risk of sudden infant death syndrome[316], and adverse effects both on the mother's health, and on the health of those with whom she shares her home[317-320]. Recent work also suggests that, over and above the effect expected by reduction of birthweight and other socioeconomic factors, educational achievement as measured at 23 years is decreased in the children of mothers who smoke[321]. Pregnancy is seen as a prime opportunity to encourage and help women to give up smoking for the benefit of their own health as well as their children's[322] with most women receiving advice on smoking from their midwives and doctors[59].

A systematic review of randomised controlled trials found that behavioural self-help approaches to smoking cessation were more effective than advice and feedback in reducing smoking in pregnancy[323] but no information was given on whether interventions were particularly helpful for disadvantaged women[324]. Cessation rates are lower in mothers from lower socioeconomic groups[59] and a survey in the West Midlands found that pregnant women on Income Support were less likely than other women to be contemplating giving up smoking[325]. Given these differences in likelihood of cessation, further development of both "upstream" (see, for example, recommendations 21 and 23) and "downstream" policies (see, for example, recommendations 26.2–26.4) are likely to be necessary to achieve a reduction in inequalities in smoking prevalence in pregnancy. Interventions that target individual behaviour alone may be insufficient[326,327].

Benefit

A decrease in prevalence in smoking during pregnancy is likely to be followed by a decrease in women who smoke after pregnancy. This should decrease smoking-related morbidity and, eventually, mortality in mothers; passive smoking-related morbidity and mortality, including sudden infant death syndrome, in those with whom she lives and works; and increased birthweight in the children of mothers who were formerly smokers, with decreases in early mortality[320]. The problems of giving up smoking for disadvantaged women are discussed elsewhere (see text for recommendations 26.2–26.4).

22.3 We recommend the further development of programmes to help women to give up smoking before or during pregnancy, and which are focused on the less well off.

Social and emotional support of parents

Inequality

Parents caring for children in disadvantaged circumstances are likely to need additional family support if they are to protect their children from the effects of disadvantage. Inequality in the need for such support is evident in the socioeconomic patterns of child abuse. Although such patterns are modified by the definition of abuse[328] and ascertainment bias[329], there is a consistent association between low socioeconomic status and child protection registrations[330]. This association is demonstrated across a range of indicators of individuals and areas, including unemployment, lone parenthood, and receipt of means-tested benefits[331-333]

Evidence

Most parents living in disadvantaged circumstances wish to, and do, protect and promote the health of their children under the most unpromising conditions[334]. A general conclusion of evaluations of family support services is that parents under stress overcome family problems more easily when there is a wide range of sources of family support available in local communities[335].

Family support enables parents under stress and children in need to have some respite from their disadvantaged circumstances, and to build protective social relationships. Family support services cover a wide range, and include neighbourhood family centres and projects, baby and child health clinics, supervised play space and day care and affordable after-school care. Consequently the Inquiry has taken the view that policies which promote the emotional and social support of parents living in circumstances of disadvantage should act at a number of different levels. These policies include those which address poverty, social isolation and lack of community resources as well as ones which provide enhanced individual or group-based support. However, the research evidence tends to be biased towards assessment of interventions to support individual parents or families, often within public service settings. This is partly because it is easier to design robust experimental evaluations of such interventions. The following section summarises this evidence, recognising that it also highlights principles relevant to community-based interventions.

Social and emotional support of parents, particularly mothers, may enhance their capacity to protect their children, especially when they are trying to do so in disadvantaged circumstances. The potency of even short periods of personal support is demonstrated by a review of the effects of continuous professional or social support during childbirth. In a number of settings, women who received support from a trained person had shorter labours, less analgesia and operative delivery, and their babies had improved APGAR scores (that is, were in better condition at birth)[306]. However, most studies have used longer periods of social support, aimed at reducing stress and enhancing self-esteem and confidence during pregnancy and the early part of parenthood. The effect of home visiting during pregnancy alone on birthweight and other pregnancy outcomes is inconsistent[334,336,337]. Some studies, whilst not showing an effect on physical health, have found social and behavioural effects. For instance, a review of controlled trials of social support in pregnancy concluded that women receiving support were less likely to feel unhappy, nervous and worried during pregnancy, and were more likely to be breastfeeding after birth[338].

Home visiting in the first 2 years of life has been associated with beneficial effects during childhood. A systematic review found that programmes of home visits by professional or specially trained lay care givers tended to be associated with decreased rates of childhood injury[339]. They may also reduce rates of child abuse, incomplete immunisations, hospital admission, and morbidity in infancy, although the evidence is not conclusive for these outcomes. The applicability of these studies to service provision in the United Kingdom is unknown. However, in the UK at least two studies have shown that appropriately trained health visitors can detect and manage postnatal depression, leading to more rapid remission of symptoms, fewer problems in the relationship between the mother and the child, and fewer child behaviour problems[340,341]. Although postnatal depression does not show a marked gradient with socioeconomic status, the long term effect of maternal depression on the cognitive and emotional behaviour of children is more marked in the presence of socioeconomic disadvantage[342].

In the UK, several experiments in home-based strategies to help parents become more self-confident and skilful in their child's development have been initiated. These have used specially trained health visitors or "community mothers", training teams of volunteers[16,343]. Early results indicate that those receiving home-based support strategies feel more positive and have higher self-esteem during early motherhood, and the children have more complete immunisations, and less early weaning onto cow's milk. Longer-term outcomes are awaited[16,344]. A systematic review of parent-training programmes in improving the behaviour of children with a behaviour disorder between 3 and 10 years concluded that group-based programmes were the most effective, although it is not known specifically which aspects of these programmes are important[345]. Such programmes might have an application in prevention as well as treatment.

Few studies have yet included long term outcomes. However, in a 15 year follow up of an American randomised controlled trial, mothers who had received home visits during pregnancy and the first 2 years after birth were less likely to have been identified as perpetrators of child abuse. Amongst those who were socioeconomically disadvantaged, those who had received home visits had fewer subsequent births, increased birth interval, received income support for a shorter period, had fewer behavioural problems associated with the use of alcohol and other drugs, and had fewer arrests[346]. A seven year follow-up in the UK has found improved health in children and mothers who had midwife-provided social support in pregnancy[347].

A number of methodological issues arise in the best way of providing parental support. The most systematically evaluated studies are the randomised controlled trials. However, these tend to be conducted in particular settings and especially in health service settings. It is not clear whether the beneficial effects observed are the consequence of a particular type of support or would be seen with the provision of any support which met the needs of parents and children even if different in content – for example, child-care or financial support – or context – for example, community-based and parent-led. In addition, the quality of support offered in an experimental setting may not be reproducible in service. Thus the nature of support, who should offer it, when, and for how long is still under debate. Secondly, the applicability to the UK of the results of studies conducted outside this country is uncertain. Thirdly, the effect on some outcomes has only been tested in single trials, and must be regarded with caution. Fourthly, the identification of those most likely to benefit from support needs to be refined. The trials have mostly been conducted amongst high-risk populations. Lastly, the best way of translating research findings based on parental empowerment into service provision which does not patronise or stigmatise users needs to be addressed[16].

Despite these issues, we have concluded that the strength of the evidence appears sufficient to recommend enhancing support for parents. Such support should be provided through policies acting at a number of different levels, including the relief of poverty (recommendation 21). Policies should be based in the community, should be family-centred and should meet the needs of families living in disadvantaged circumstances. In the spirit of the Children Act (1989), they should include further development of services provided on the basis of partnership with parents and between agencies[328,348].

Health visitors already aim to provide social and emotional support to parents and are acceptable to mothers in disadvantaged settings[349,350]. We consider that an enhancement of their role and capacity to provide social and emotional support of disadvantaged parents is needed, as part of the range of neighbourhood services to support parents.

Benefit

Increased social and emotional support of parents should reduce the impact of disadvantage and enhance parenting skills, with consequent social and behavioural gains in health for their children. It should also enhance self-esteem in parents. A range of other physical, social and mental health gains are possible in both parents and children. None of the evidence points to harm from support of parents, but this pre-supposes that services are delivered in an enabling and non-stigmatising manner.

23. We RECOMMEND policies that promote the social and emotional support for parents and children. Specifically:

23.1 we recommend the further development of the role and capacity of health visitors to provide social and emotional support to expectant parents, and parents with young children.

Promoting the health of looked-after children

Our recommendations on the support of families are aimed at promoting child and parental health and at the prevention of child abuse and family dysfunction. We recognise the necessity of recommending policies which will address the health needs of children who are "looked-after" by local authorities.

There were about 89,000 children looked-after by social service departments in England at any time during the year ending in March 1997, with about 65 per cent in foster placements[330]. Looked-after children are at particular risk of both early life and later disadvantage[333]. More than 75 per cent of looked-after children leave care with no educational qualifications and between 50 per cent and 80 per cent of care-leavers are unemployed[351]. It is estimated that 30 per cent of young single homeless people have been in care. High rates of alcohol use and cigarette smoking are also reported among care-leavers and it is estimated that one in seven young women leaving care are either pregnant or already mothers[352]. Children with an experience of public care are also vulnerable to substance misuse and mental health problems in adult life[353,354].

This cluster of socioeconomic and health disadvantage means that looked-after children are a key target group for policies related to education, employment and housing, and to health related behaviour, recommended earlier in our report. However, they are further disadvantaged in their access to health care, both preventative and therapeutic. Their increased mobility may result in fragmentation of, and delay in, service delivery, including assessment of, and provision for, their educational and health needs, including health promotion.

Looked-after children lack a professional advocate for their health. We recommend that looked-after children have a designated medical adviser to identify their physical and psychological health needs, and negotiate service delivery. However, this alone is unlikely to be sufficient. Looked-after children tend not to respond to health information and effective ways of providing them with appropriate information need to be further developed[355].

23.2 We recommend local authorities identify and address the physical and psychological health needs of looked-after children.

8. Young People and Adults of Working Age

This section sets out inequalities in the health of young people and adults of working age. It summarises the evidence which we have concluded indicates areas for future policy development, and the benefits which may result from such policies. Many recommendations given already will apply to this group. In particular, work is an important determinant of health inequalities at this stage of the life course.

We recommend policies which improve the opportunities for work and which ameliorate the health consequences of unemployment (recommendation 8).

We recommend policies to improve the quality of jobs, and reduce psychosocial work hazards (recommendation 9).

Our additional recommendations relate to preventing suicide, particularly in young men and people who are known to be mentally ill, and promoting the adoption of healthy lifestyles.

Preventing suicide

Inequality

Suicide is more common in men than in women, and in lower socioeconomic groups. In 1996 the rates were three times higher for males than females. The highest rates are for men aged 25–44 and those over 75 years[25]. In 1991–1993 (the most recent data available by social class) in England and Wales, mortality from suicide for men was 4 times greater in social class V than in social class I[29]. The international literature consistently shows higher rates of suicide in young south Asian women, whilst lower rates are found in African Americans and African Caribbeans[356]. The overall age-standardised mortality rate for suicide has fallen by nearly a half in women over the last 20 years, but has hardly changed for men. This hides the information that over the same period, for men under 44, there has been a rise of 20–30 per cent whereas for men aged 45 and over there has been a fall of about the same magnitude[32].

Evidence

Suicide is associated with unemployment, alcohol and substance misuse, imprisonment, and mental disorder[357]. Up to half of all people who commit suicide have a history of self-harm, and up to 1 per cent of people who self-harm go on to kill themselves[358-360]. People who deliberately self-harm are also likely to have problems with a relationship, employment, education, alcohol, substance misuse, and/or finances[361].

Policies to prevent suicide include those aimed at the causes of social exclusion which may lead to suicide. These include: social support for parents (recommendation 23); pre-school education (recommendation 5); the development of "life skills" and the prevention of alcohol and substance misuse (recommendation 6); provision of adequate housing (recommendation 10, 11 and 12); the relief of poverty and reduction of unemployment (recommendation 8); the promotion of healthy workplaces (recommendation 9); and policies which promote social cohesion.

The association of suicide with existing mental illness suggests that policies for the care of young people with mental illness also provide opportunities for the prevention of suicide. About a quarter of those who kill themselves have been in contact with specialist mental health services in the year before their deaths[362]. A recent review on the promotion of mental health in high-risk groups reinforces the role of the primary health-care team both in identifying and co-ordinating the management of people at high risk[363]. Community mental health teams may be more effective than non-team standard care in preventing suicide in those who are already severely mentally ill[364]. Both types of team, which may have considerable overlap, need to ensure effective working between different disciplines and agencies[363]. An important component of the work of such teams is to address all the needs of the patient, including employment, housing and social support. Furthermore, particular strategies may be required to meet the needs of young people who either cannot or do not choose to access current services. These include people who default from follow up, absent themselves from school, or are in prison or young offenders' institutions.

Benefit

Most policies recommended here are aimed at the improvement of socioeconomic and living conditions, and social cohesion. They will have many benefits in addition to their contribution to the prevention of suicide.

24. *We RECOMMEND measures to prevent suicide among young people, especially among young men and seriously mentally ill people.*

Promoting healthier lifestyles

Health related behaviour is an important determinant of health and inequalities in health. However, the reasons why individuals adopt one form of behaviour rather than another are complex. They include the influence of earlier experience, including that as a very young child, the social and economic environment, work or school, and the cultural milieu, as well as characteristics specific to the individual. Furthermore the effects of health related behaviour or its consequences differ between individuals and between groups, depending on their susceptibility to these influences. For example the effect of a high body mass index in adult life on blood pressure is greater in people who were of lower birthweight[301].

Thus, policies designed to change health related behaviour need to act at different levels, and to accept that behaviour change, for instance in the changing of children's dietary habits, may take some time to become apparent. The Inquiry considers that, as with inequalities in health in general, inequalities in health related behaviours need to be approached on a broad front considering both "upstream" and "downstream" policies, and policies which cover both short and longer-term benefits. This section sets out inequalities in health related behaviour and the evidence which we have concluded indicates areas for future policy development. Many of the more "upstream" policies in this area have been considered earlier in this report, and are cross-referenced. However, we wish to emphasise that these "upstream" policies are of crucial importance in reducing inequalities in health related behaviour. Furthermore, we consider that policies aimed at changing health related behaviour should avoid attaching blame or stigma to individuals or groups. Thus our recommendations are based on the principles of increasing information and choice to individuals and communities, and enabling them to make healthy choices[365].

Promoting sexual health

Inequality

Men and women from manual households have a median age at first intercourse about 2 years lower than for those from social class I households. Black young people are more likely to have first intercourse under the age of 16 than white or Asian young people. The proportions with first intercourse under the age of 16 are 26 per cent for Black men, and 10 per cent for Black women, compared to 19 per cent and 8 per cent for young white people and 11 per cent and 1 per cent for young Asian people[366].

Under-age conception rates for places within Britain are highly correlated with indices of deprivation, with high rates in areas which are deprived[260]. However, the relatively small number of events makes further analysis difficult. There is a fourfold difference between the health authorities with the highest and lowest rates, and large differences between one time period and another.

Evidence

For many young women, pregnancy and motherhood are positive and welcomed experiences without long term negative outcomes. However, compared to women aged 20 to 35 years, teenage mothers and their children are at higher risk of experiencing adverse health, educational, social and economic outcomes[130]. Approximately half of the pregnancies in under 16 year olds and a third of those in 16–19 year olds are terminated[260]. These terminations, along with miscarriages, can also have an adverse effect on the health of teenagers.

The risk of teenage pregnancy is increased in association with a number of social, socioeconomic and individual factors, many of which are more common in people experiencing disadvantage – for example, low educational attainment, poor housing. Particularly at risk are the daughters of teenage mothers, young people "looked-after" by the local authority or leaving care, school non-attendees – due to truancy or exclusion – and homeless or runaway teenagers. Although it is difficult to establish cause and effect, it is possible that reducing inequalities in some of these socioeconomic risk factors – for example, poverty or educational attainment – would reduce inequalities in unwanted teenage pregnancy[130].

More specific interventions to promote sexual health focus on education and provision of appropriate and sensitive contraceptive services[130]. Features associated with successful sex education programmes include: timing, which should precede the onset of sexual activity; a combined approach to education and information about the provision of contraception; integration with psychological approaches, and with other life management skills; context, emphasising responsible and caring relationships and a recognition of social influences and pressures; a focus on specific aims, such as delayed intercourse and safe intercourse; and the tailoring of the programmes to the needs of the group they are intended to serve[129,130].

Most of the evaluated programmes have focused on addressing individual factors associated with teenage pregnancy, rather than the associated social and economic factors. No studies have specifically focused on reduction of inequalities in risk of outcomes. The role of sex education is discussed earlier in the text supporting recommendation 6 on the development of health promoting schools.

The role of parents in sex education also needs to be recognised. Under the age of about 16 years young people generally report that their parents should be the main source of information about sex but in practice this is often not the case. Appropriate means to help parents increase their skills and confidence in sex education need to be developed. The media also have an important role to play in providing information and influencing the climate of opinion[367].

Provision of contraceptive services to teenagers is highly cost effective, saving £377 and £466 per unwanted pregnancy avoided for clinic and general practice provision respectively, even if only the resource consequences for the NHS of pregnancy are taken into account. The savings are much greater if the longer term health gains are considered[130]. However, teenagers may lack information about contraceptive use or availability. A recent review of the literature found a lack of UK evidence on the effectiveness or cost effectiveness of different approaches to the delivery of contraceptive services to young people. Descriptive studies suggest that services should be based on a local needs assessment and ensure accessibility and confidentiality. Clinic-based settings may be used more than those in primary care. Because of the nature of teenagers' sexual activity, which can be unplanned and sporadic, provision of emergency contraception is important. However, there is widespread public and professional misunderstanding of the use of emergency contraception, which may merit particular health education action[130].

Interventions have not evaluated whether policies will preferentially promote sexual health and reduce unwanted teenage pregnancy rates in people experiencing disadvantage. Targeting of education on contraceptive provision – for example, by individual characteristics or by area – might be a way of reducing inequalities. Over half of teenage pregnancies continue to delivery. Policies and evidence on preventing the adverse health and social outcomes of teenage pregnancy are presented under recommendations 21 and 23.

Benefit

For more "upstream" policies, promotion of sexual health and prevention of unwanted pregnancy might be only some of many benefits. In general, sex education programmes have not been associated with increased sexual activity or its complications and some have been associated with delayed onset of sexual activity[129,130]. Sex education and appropriate contraceptive use are likely to decrease rates of sexually transmitted diseases and promote other aspects of sexual health. Prevention of unwanted teenage pregnancy will reduce the risks to the physical, mental and social health of the potential mother.

25. We RECOMMEND policies which promote sexual health in young people and reduce unwanted teenage pregnancy, including access to appropriate contraceptive services.

Encouraging physical exercise

Inequality

Levels of physical activity in men show a complex pattern with social class, with more men in lower social classes reporting physical activity as part of their occupation and more men in higher social classes reporting moderate or vigorous walking and leisure activity. In women there are similar gradients in walking and leisure activity and no clear pattern with occupational activity. People in lower socioeconomic groups walk more than those in higher groups but are less likely to describe their walking pace as brisk or fast. Inactivity, which may be a better predictor of obesity, is more common in lower social classes for both men and women[35].

The proportion of men who are obese has risen from 13 per cent in 1993 to 16 per cent in 1996. For women the equivalent figures are 16 per cent and 18 per cent. Obesity is higher in the lower social classes in women, with 25 per cent in class V being classified as obese compared to 14 per cent in social class I and with intermediate proportions in the classes between I and V. In men, there are lower rates of obesity in social class I (11 per cent) but the higher rates in social class V (18 per cent) are similar to those in the remaining classes[37]. Rates of obesity and mean body mass index appear to be increasing for school-aged children[368].

Evidence

Increased physical activity of moderate intensity is associated with lower overall mortality rates and decreased risks of mortality from cardiovascular disease, colon cancer and non-insulin dependent diabetes mellitus. Regular physical activity prevents or delays the development of hypertension, and reduces blood pressure in those with hypertension. These effects may be, in part, mediated by the fact that physical activity prevents weight gain and obesity. Physical activity also relieves the symptoms of depression and anxiety and is important in the prevention of osteoporosis. As these are common conditions, relatively small reductions in risk of them would result in significant gains in public health[369-372].

Recommendations to promote moderate intensity exercise most commonly cite brisk walking as the mode of physical activity[373]. Walking is the most common form of physical activity across all socioeconomic groups, although both the number of journeys undertaken on foot and the annual average distance walked are decreasing[236,259]. Interventions where the mode of exercise being promoted is walking appear to be more effective than those that depend on attending a special facility to practice games or sports[374]. Walking should also be more accessible to those in lower socioeconomic groups, as it does not require costly equipment or training. In addition it can, theoretically, be incorporated into everyday routines, although in deprived areas, improved access to a safe and pleasant environment would be a necessary pre-condition. The provision of low-cost keep fit classes in existing local facilities, such as community centres or schools is one option.

Most interventions have been tested on white, middle-aged, well-educated men and women, and it is not known whether interventions would differentially benefit those in lower socioeconomic groups. The relative effectiveness of different types of intervention is largely unknown.

The evidence on encouraging walking and cycling and the safe separation of pedestrians and cyclists from motor vehicles is given in the text for recommendation 15. These policies may be particularly important in promoting exercise in children.

Fear of accidents and harm is an important component in the increasing use of transport of children in cars, particularly to and from school. The promotion of physical activity, over and above participation in formal physical education, is one of the roles of health promotion within schools (see recommendation 6).

Benefit

Decreased levels of inactivity and increased physical activity should reduce and prevent obesity, cardiovascular disease and non-insulin dependent diabetes mellitus. As well as these health benefits, opportunities afforded by exercise might also lead to wider social networks and increased social cohesion.

Reducing tobacco smoking

Inequality

There is a higher prevalence of cigarette smoking in lower socioeconomic groups. In 1996, 29 per cent of men and 28 per cent of women smoked but this ranged from 2 per cent of men (11% of women) in professional occupations to 41 per cent men (36 per cent of women) in unskilled manual occupations. Amongst smokers, men and women in professional occupations smoke fewer cigarettes per week than those in unskilled manual occupations[28]. Furthermore, nicotine dependence is higher in people experiencing disadvantage, with higher plasma cotinine levels even after adjusting for the number of cigarettes smoked[35,37]. Not only do men and women in the lower groups have higher prevalence rates, they also have lower cessation rates. Since 1973 rates of cessation have more than doubled in the most advantaged groups, from 25 per cent to over 50 per cent. In the least well off groups, there has been a very limited increase in cessation rates from 8 to 9 per cent cessation in 1973 to 10 to 13 per cent in 1996[375].

Evidence

Smoking is an important component of differences in mortality between social classes[376]. In the United Kingdom, more cancer deaths can be attributed to smoking tobacco than to any other single risk factor. In 1995, smoking was estimated to account for more than 30,000 deaths from lung cancer, and a further 16,000 deaths from cancer of other sites, notably the oesophagus, bladder, stomach, mouth and throat, contributing to approximately one third of the mortality of cancer as a whole[377]. Smoking is also an important cause of chronic obstructive lung disease, coronary heart disease, stroke and aortic aneurysm. Furthermore, smoking damages the health of non-smokers. A recent review concluded that passive smoking causes lung cancer and coronary heart disease in adult non-smokers, and respiratory disease, sudden infant death syndrome, middle ear disease and asthmatic attacks in children[320].

For the population as a whole, tobacco consumption falls when the real price of tobacco rises[378–380]. The price elasticity of cigarettes is higher among young people.

Studies in the United States and Canada indicate that young people's intention to smoke and their uptake of smoking are highly price-sensitive[381-386]. An important factor in explaining the greater effect of price on young people is that most are not habitual, nicotine dependent, smokers. Price rises can therefore be an effective way of preventing the onset of regular smoking in adolescence. With very few smokers taking up regular smoking after the age of 20, price can clearly have a longer-term impact on the prevalence of smoking and thus on inequalities in smoking-related disease.

However the real price of tobacco has a disproportionate effect on the living standards of Britain's poorest households, for whom expenditure on tobacco is a larger proportion of disposable income[387]. Households in the lowest tenth of income spend 6 times as much of their income on tobacco as households in the highest tenth[278]. Over 70 per cent of two-parent households on Income Support buy cigarettes, spending about 15 per cent of their disposable income on tobacco[388]. Approximately 55 per cent of lone mothers on Income Support smoke, smoking on average 5 packets of cigarettes per week[327]. Studies of the cost of meeting basic needs, which explicitly exclude spending on tobacco, indicate that Income Support levels are insufficient to secure a basic but adequate standard of living, especially if the households contain children[65,78,81,84,85]. Not surprisingly, therefore, low income households where the parents smoke are much more likely to be lacking basic amenities, including food, shoes and coats than non-smoking parents on Income Support[388].

Although smoking prevalence has decreased overall, despite increases in the real price of tobacco, it has remained stable amongst people who are most disadvantaged[375]. A recent longitudinal survey of lone mothers found that living in severe hardship was the primary deterrent to quitting. This makes it unlikely that increasing the price of tobacco, and so decreasing disposable income and increasing hardship, will increase cessation rates in disadvantaged households[327].

Advertising bans in Canada and New Zealand have reduced tobacco consumption. We note that the European Union Council of Ministers formally adopted the Directive to ban tobacco advertising and sponsorship in May 1998. Media advocacy and creation of unpaid publicity may not result directly in cessation but form the basis of public opinion on which other measures rest. Restrictions on smoking in public places or the workplace probably reduce consumption but the effects on cessation are undetermined. However, they may reduce the effects of passive smoking. Overall, evidence does not indicate which policies are the most effective in reducing inequalities[320,380]. The relatively stable rate of cessation in disadvantaged groups over the last 20 years suggests that simply intensifying current approaches is unlikely to sufficient.

The cultural and environmental barriers that disadvantaged people face in quitting smoking will take time to change. In the shorter term, a complementary strategy is to reduce nicotine dependence, which is likely to be stronger in disadvantaged smokers than amongst the affluent[35,37].

Nicotine replacement therapy (NRT) has been shown to be an effective treatment aid, approximately doubling success rates from both brief and intensive treatments, and with evidence that its efficacy is maintained in real world settings[389-393]. It is not known whether it is preferentially effective in helping those who are disadvantaged to quit. Trials have found that NRT is effective in helping nicotine-dependent smokers to stop smoking[390,393]. Because there is a socioeconomic gradient in nicotine dependence, NRT may therefore have a differentially beneficial effect in smokers in lower socioeconomic groups. However, as it is currently sold at commercial rates over the counter, its price could prohibit its use amongst people on low incomes[394]. Preliminary evidence suggests better compliance and outcome when the smoker does not have to pay[395]. NRT could be made available on prescription or through other mechanisms which make it free to those who are least able to afford it[394,396]. NRT on prescription would also have the benefit of involving general practitioners in smoking cessation. Brief advice from a general practitioner is a highly cost effective method of promoting cessation of smoking, with cessation rates equivalent to rates achieved as a result of mass media campaigns, up to 5 per cent[380]. Community-based interventions and specialised smoking clinics are also effective settings in which to provide NRT[390].

Benefit

Reduction in smoking would decrease the risk of smoking related diseases over a period of time and decrease the risks of passive smoking to companions in various settings. The relative differences in mortality by socioeconomic group are similar in smokers and non-smokers. However, given the higher mortality rate in smokers and the increased rates of smoking in lower socioeconomic groups, reduction in smoking in all socioeconomic groups will decrease the absolute difference in mortality rates between socioeconomic groups[277].

Reducing alcohol-related harm

Inequality

Deaths from diseases caused by alcohol show a clear gradient with socioeconomic position, with an almost fourfold higher rate in unskilled working men compared to those from professional groups. In addition, alcohol is a contributory factor to deaths from accidents, which also show a pronounced socioeconomic gradient[397].

Amongst people under the age of 30 years, there is little variation in consumption of alcohol by socioeconomic group. However problem drinking is twice as common in the poorest as in the most affluent, 17 per cent versus 8 per cent for men and 6 per cent versus 3 per cent for women. In older adults, a similar pattern exists for men. In older women consumption is greater in the affluent, but there is no socioeconomic gradient in problem drinking, and poor women are more likely than the affluent to report being drunk[35]. Higher levels of consumption of alcohol have been consistently observed in some deprived groups, such as unemployed people[398-400] and those who are homeless[401,402]. These observations suggest that the pattern of drinking influences alcohol-related health inequalities. Problem drinking is associated with delinquency, criminality and violence, including domestic violence and child abuse. The degree to which health-damaging drinking patterns in young people persist into later life is unclear. Deprivation may contribute to the probability of continuing to drink in a hazardous fashion, and may also inhibit opportunities for positive changes in behaviour. Heavy drinking in people in higher socioeconomic groups may be less harmful than in lower socioeconomic groups because they are protected from harmful effects by better diet, housing, health care and other factors[403].

Evidence

At a population level, there is a positive correlation between mean consumption and the prevalence of heavy drinking. This suggests that one mechanism to reduce problem drinking and thus alcohol-related harm, is to reduce mean consumption[404]. Overall population consumption is affected by price[405–407]. Increasing the price of alcohol may decrease consumption amongst low income problem drinkers but the effect of price elasticity on different groups has been little studied[408,409].

Problem drinking in young people may be influenced by wider measures which support them and enhance their chances of employment and improved living conditions. Sensible drinking habits may be engendered in childhood and so be affected by interventions at school (see recommendation 6).

A reduction in the permitted level of blood alcohol concentration for driving from 80 to 50 mg/100 ml has been associated with reduced rates of alcohol-related accidents and risk behaviour in some countries[410]. The introduction of random breath testing is another option which may be a significant deterrent to drinking and driving[410,411]. The provision of adequate and affordable transport would assist in reducing the perceived need to drive after drinking.

People with alcohol-related problems who are disadvantaged in other ways, through having limited financial or social resources or being homeless, may have less access to appropriate treatment services for all their needs, including treatment of their alcohol-related health problems[196–199]. Recommendation 11 addresses this inequity.

Benefit

A decrease in problem drinking should reduce alcohol-related disease and accidents, as well as some types of anti-social behaviour.

26. We RECOMMEND policies which promote the adoption of healthier lifestyles, particularly in respect of factors which show a strong social gradient in prevalence or consequences. Specifically:

26.1 we recommend policies which promote moderate intensity exercise including: further provision of cycling and walking routes to school, and other environmental modifications aimed at the safe separation of pedestrians and cyclists from motor vehicles; and safer opportunities for leisure.

26.2 We recommend policies to reduce tobacco smoking including: restricting smoking in public places; abolishing tobacco advertising and promotion; and community, mass media and educational initiatives.

26.3 We recommend increases in the real price of tobacco to discourage young people from becoming habitual smokers and to encourage adult smokers to quit. These increases should be introduced in tandem with policies to improve the living standards of low income households and policies to help smokers in these households become and remain ex-smokers.

26.4 We recommend making nicotine replacement therapy available on prescription.

26.5 We recommend policies which reduce alcohol-related ill health, accidents and violence, including measures which at least maintain the real cost of alcohol.

9. Older people

In this section, older people are defined as those aged 65 years or over, unless stated otherwise.

Inequality

Mortality data by social class are limited in older people, because occupation is not recorded at all on the death certificates of men or women over the age of 75 years and is recorded for married women only if the woman has been in paid work for the majority of her life. Thus, alternative measures of social classification, such as housing tenure, are needed to describe socioeconomic differences in mortality in older people. Compared to the national average, the mortality rates in people aged 60 to 74 who had been living in local authority rented accommodation showed a 16 per cent excess, whereas rates for people who had been living in owner occupied accommodation showed a 13–14 per cent deficit[412]. Although data are available on fewer specific causes of death than in younger cohorts, patterns seem to be similar after the age of 65 years. The most pronounced differences between socioeconomic groups are for lung cancer and respiratory disease, coronary heart disease and stroke, all of which show higher rates as disadvantage increases [30,412,413]. Life expectancy at age 65 years is 2.6 years greater in men (2 years greater in women) from social classes I and II compared to men from classes IV and V[31].

Prevention of morbidity and disability rather than mortality may be a more relevant focus in older people. Available data, which are fewer than those for younger age groups, suggest that older people experiencing disadvantage tend to have poor health. Respiratory function is lower and blood pressure higher in people from lower socioeconomic groups[37]. Older people from lower socioeconomic groups have higher rates of total tooth loss than those from higher socioeconomic groups[414]. Long standing illness prevalence is greater in unskilled manual groups of men over the age of 65 years than in men from professional groups, 72 per cent and 53 per cent respectively. However, there is no corresponding difference for women[28].

The following sections set out specific inequalities in the health and socioeconomic determinants of health in older people, and summarise the evidence which we have concluded indicates areas for future policy development to reduce these inequalities. These areas are: promoting the material well-being of older people; improving the quality of their homes; promoting the maintenance of mobility, independence and social contacts; and improving health and social services. The sections on each also indicate the benefit which may result from such policies. The inequalities, evidence and benefit in relation to most of these policies have been discussed in earlier parts of this report. They are raised again in brief here, with particular regard to their relevance for older people. As the majority of older people are women, and the ratio of women to men increases with age, some areas are discussed again in the section on gender.

Promoting material well-being

Inequality

Older people are more likely to be living in poverty, whether this is defined as below half-average income or the receipt of means-tested benefits[65]. This is particularly true for older women. There are three times as many female as male recipients of Income Support[77].

Evidence

The poorest pensioners, who rely most on benefit, have experienced a relative deterioration in their income. This is the result of cutting the link between increases in earnings and annual rises in pensions and benefits in the 1980s. Current levels of pensions are not generous compared to other European Union countries[79]. Older people are at risk of fuel poverty[96,97], and may face extra costs in purchasing social and health care. Disabled pensioner households are more likely to be reliant on state benefits than non-disabled pensioner households[415].

Around one million state retirement pensioners do not take up the means-tested benefits to which they are entitled, losing on average £16 per week[86,87]. A number of factors may operate, including lack of knowledge of entitlement, a perception of being stigmatised by the receipt of benefit, and physical or other difficulties in the processes of claiming. Possible ways of overcoming some of these problems are the establishment of new organisations or agencies: a separate pensioners' agency[88]; a citizens' bank[88]; or a welfare counsellor in primary care[89]. Schemes such as welfare counselling in primary care could also raise awareness of other entitlements, for instance free dentures. Fear of cost is thought to deter some poor older people from seeking services and aids which would, in fact, be free to them[416–419].

Benefit

Measures which increase the income of poor older people are likely to improve their living standards, such as promoting better nutrition and heating, and so lead to improvements in health.

27. We RECOMMEND policies which will promote the material well being of older people. Specifically:

we recommend policies which will further reduce income inequalities, and improve the living standards of households in receipt of social security benefits (recommendation 3).

We recommend uprating of benefits and pensions according to principles which protect and, where possible, improve the standard of living of those who depend on them and which narrow the gap between their standard of living and average living standards (recommendation 3.2).

We recommend measures to increase the uptake of benefits among entitled groups (recommendation 3.3).

Improving the quality of homes

Inequality

Properties in poor condition are disproportionately occupied by single older people, and tend to be older, privately rented properties[209]. Older women are particularly likely to live alone[420,421].

Evidence

Unmodernised homes have high heating costs. Cold housing leads directly to hypothermia and may contribute to the excess of winter deaths seen in older people[208,215]. It also leads to fuel poverty[96,97]. Schemes which aim to improve insulation and heating efficiency are the most direct way of addressing this problem. Poor housing design contributes to major accidents in older people and seemingly minor accidents which may have grave consequences[208]. Home visits for the assessment and modification of hazards can reduce falls in older people[422].

Benefit

Removal of hazards in the home is likely to lead to reduced death and injury from accidents. Improvements in home design may allow older disabled people to be cared for at home, with improvements in their quality of life.

28. We RECOMMEND the quality of homes in which older people live be improved. Specifically:

we recommend policies to improve insulation and heating systems in new and existing buildings in order to further reduce the prevalence of fuel poverty (recommendation 12.1).

We recommend amending housing and licensing conditions and housing regulations on space and amenity to reduce accidents in the home, including measures to promote the installation of smoke detectors in existing homes (recommendation 12.2).

Promoting the maintenance of mobility, independence, and social contacts

Inequality

Lack of access to transport is experienced disproportionately by older people[229], limiting their access to goods, services, opportunities and social contacts[423,424]. This is particularly a problem for older women[40,282] and older people who are disabled[425]. Older people are more likely to fear becoming victims of crime than younger people. This restricts their opportunities to leave their homes, particularly at night[220].

Evidence

High traffic volumes result in feelings of insecurity[234] and decrease walking as well as the use of other transport[426,427]. The use of public transport is partly determined by price[238,239]. There are over 10 million older people who are eligible for concessionary fares. Concessionary fare schemes vary from place to place[258] and in places are very limited. Furthermore, uptake of concessions is lower in areas of low population density, and only 39 per cent in rural areas[259].

Benefit

Greater opportunity for travel through the availability of affordable and effective public transport should remove a barrier to health-promoting opportunities. For example improved access to community based leisure facilities, which might include the facilities of health promoting schools, should allow increased opportunity for older people to enjoy physical and social activity. Increased exercise is important in preserving muscle tone. This decreases the risk of falling and thus injury, and reduces the disability caused by osteoarthritis.

29. We RECOMMEND policies which will promote the maintenance of mobility, independence, and social contacts. Specifically:

we recommend the development of policies to reduce the fear of crime and violence, and to create a safe environment for people to live in (recommendation 13).

We recommend the further development of a high quality public transport system which is integrated with other forms of transport and is affordable to the user (recommendation 14).

We recommend concessionary fares should be available to pensioners and disadvantaged groups throughout the country, and that local schemes should emulate high quality schemes, such as those of London and the West Midlands (recommendation 18).

Improving services

Inequality

Poor older people may be less likely to receive some health care services[428,429], or may have poorer health outcome after receiving these services[428]. For instance severe visual problems are more likely to remain unrecognised and untreated in older people from low socioeconomic groups[430,431].

Evidence

Functional capacity relies on sight, hearing, mobility and continence. Older people from low socioeconomic groups have higher rates of ill health and disability than those from more affluent groups. Health and social services can ameliorate the experience of poor health and disability in old age, and should be accessible and distributed on the basis of need. However, levels of domiciliary support are insufficient to counter an increasing trend for more older people to enter residential care[425].

Although data are sparse, user fees – for instance for sight tests or dentures – may deter poor older people from seeking services[416-419]. Where demand for services exceeds supply, such as for social services support – home cleaning, shopping, bathing and meals – user fees may disadvantage those below average income, even if the poorest groups are protected through means-testing. Furthermore, poorer older people are less able to bear the additional costs of disability, such as the additional laundry costs associated with incontinence. Whenever a significant private sector exists, for instance in chiropody, poorer older people are likely to have decreased access[428].

There has been considerable discussion on whether "ageism" exists within health services[428,432]. Ageism in this context means the withholding of beneficial care, on the basis of the person's age. The Inquiry has not considered inequalities in health (or health care) by age group to be within its terms of reference. However, we consider that services should be provided on the basis of need, and that age alone should not be a reason for withholding a service.

Benefit

By definition, services distributed in relation to need will result in health gain, which will be greatest in those most in need.

30. We RECOMMEND the further development of health and social services for older people, so that these services are accessible and distributed according to need.

Monitoring inequalities

Inequalities in health that are demonstrable earlier in life persist throughout the lifespan into old age[428]. However, there is a lack of routinely collected reliable data on social class or other markers of socioeconomic status in people after the age of retirement. This leads to particular problems in monitoring inequalities in health and its determinants in older people.

We recommend a review of data needs to improve the capacity to monitor inequalities in health and their determinants at a national and local level (recommendation 1.2).

10. Ethnicity

Ethnicity is difficult to define, but most definitions reflect self-identification with cultural traditions that provide both a meaningful social identity and boundaries between groups[433]. In this section we have considered evidence which uses various definitions of ethnicity. However, in the main these definitions are those which people apply to themselves. Thus ethnicity as used here includes cultural identity, place of origin and skin colour, and so includes white and non-white groups. Because country of birth rather than ethnic group is recorded on death certificates, mortality data are restricted to migrants only.

In the 1991 Census just over 3 million people, 5.5 per cent of the population, identified themselves as belonging to one of the non-white minority ethnic groups. Almost half had been born in the United Kingdom[434]. White minority ethnic groups were not counted on Census night. However recent estimates show that the Irish form the largest minority ethnic group, comprising 4.6 per cent of the population[435]. Data collected at the 1991 Census show that people from minority ethnic groups are more likely to live in South East England (especially London), the West Midlands, West Yorkshire and Greater Manchester. These places are home to 75 per cent of the minority ethnic population compared to only 25 per cent of the majority population[434,436].

The age and gender distribution of minority ethnic groups is different from the majority population. Some minority ethnic groups have more men than women, and all are relatively young[437]. African Caribbean and South Asian communities have a higher proportion of households with children than the white population. Around 3 in 10 households with a white head of household contain children under the age of 16 years. Comparable figures for minority ethnic groups are over 4 in 10 for African Caribbean households, 5 in 10 for Indian households and 8 in 10 for Bangladeshi and Pakistani households. Pakistani and Bangladeshi families also have more children than families in the majority white population, whilst African Caribbean, Indian and Chinese families have similar numbers of children. Pakistani and Bangladeshi households are also larger because they are more likely to have 3 or more adults, whilst African Caribbean households are more likely to be headed by a lone parent[66,438].

Inequality

Country of birth rather than ethnic group is recorded on death certificates. Thus mortality data presented below are restricted to migrants, but include migrants from Scotland, Northern Ireland and the Republic of Ireland.

Mortality

In 1989–92 mortality ratios for deaths, including perinatal mortality, from all causes for nearly all migrant groups were higher than average. However, those born in the Caribbean had a lower than average mortality ratio. For each group, except women born in Scotland, mortality from all causes fell between 1971 and 1991[61]. Cause and age specific mortality varies by country of birth. For instance, mortality from coronary heart disease is higher than average for people born in South Asia, Ireland and Scotland and lower than average for those born in the Caribbean and men born in West Africa. Mortality ratios for cerebrovascular disease are significantly higher than the average for all migrant groups except those born in East Africa. By contrast, mortality ratios for lung cancer are low in migrant groups born in the Caribbean, Asia and Africa and high in people born in Scotland or Ireland, whereas cervical cancer mortality is high for women born in the Caribbean[61,439,440]. Mortality from suicide is also unusually high in young South Asian women born in India[356]. Mortality ratios for accidents in people under the age of 15 years and over the age of 65 years are greater in migrants from Ireland and the Indian sub-continent than those born in England and Wales[252].

Morbidity

This section uses self identified ethnic group as the basis of analysis. Due to lack of data, unless stated otherwise white minority groups are included in "whites".

Overall people from minority ethnic groups are more likely to describe their health as "fair" or "poor" than the ethnic majority, although this difference comes from the poorer self-reported health of Pakistani and Bangladeshi people, and, to a lesser extent, African Caribbean people[441]. Chinese people consult less with their general practitioner (GP) than whites and African Asians are as likely to have consulted with their GP as whites. All other groups consult more[441].

A variety of conditions show differences between ethnic groups. For example, South Asians have a tendency to central obesity and insulin resistance which may pre-dispose them to diabetes and coronary heart disease[442]. On the other hand, African Caribbean people have low death rates from coronary heart disease despite their high prevalence of diabetes and hypertension[61]. Depression appears to be more common in African Caribbeans than in whites[441]. Tuberculosis is more common in Pakistanis, Bangladeshis and Black Africans than in whites, and the incidence of tuberculosis in these groups is rising[443].

There are limited data on morbidity in white minority ethnic groups, and they were included with the white majority in the Fourth National Survey of Ethnic Minorities, the source of much of the recent data on the health of minority ethnic groups. However available data support the view that Irish people have higher rates of morbidity as well as mortality. Analysis of the long standing illness question in the Census, for example, shows rates are higher for those born in Ireland[444]. Rates of hospital admission for psychiatric disorder are also high in Irish people[445].

Smoking is more common in African Caribbean and Bangladeshi men where the rates of smoking (42 per cent and 49 per cent) exceed those in white men (34 per cent). Indian and African Asian men report the lowest rates (19 per cent and 22 per cent). By contrast, in women rates of smoking are low (5 per cent or less) for all groups, except African Caribbean women, where the rates (31 per cent) are similar to those in white women (37 per cent). Alcohol consumption tends to be lower in all minority ethnic groups for both men and women compared to that in the white population. Comparable information is lacking for Scots and Irish people living in England and Wales. Total abstinence is common amongst Muslim groups, predominantly within the Pakistani and Bangladeshi communities[441].

In a survey of reported physical activity fewer men and women aged 16 to 74 years from minority ethnic groups than from the general population reported levels of activity which would benefit their health (defined as at least 30 minutes of moderate intensity physical activity on at least five days per week). For instance, amongst South Asian men aged 16 to 74 years, 67 per cent of Indians, 72 per cent of Pakistanis, and 75 per cent of Bangladeshis reported that they did not take part in enough physical activity to benefit their health, compared with 59 per cent of men in the general population. For South Asian women, the corresponding figures were 83, 86 and 82 per cent compared with 68 per cent of women in the general population. Furthermore, men and women from minority ethnic groups were more likely to report being sedentary than men and women from the general population[446].

Socioeconomic status

(Due to lack of data, unless stated otherwise white minority groups are included in "whites".)

There are important differences between ethnic groups in factors which are associated with health, and which the Inquiry has taken the view are determinants of health. Firstly, socioeconomic status is different between ethnic groups. Compared to the majority white population (unemployment rate 6.5 per cent), Labour Force Survey estimates of rates of male unemployment are slightly higher in Indians (7.4 per cent), and considerably higher in African Caribbean (20.5 per cent), and Pakistani and Bangladeshi groups (15.9 per cent)[45]. The sample size is too small for reliable estimates of rates in Chinese people. Surveys of minority ethnic groups have higher absolute percentages of people out of work, but the same pattern of differences between groups[66,441]. Part of these differences is due to the relatively young average age of these minority ethnic groups, and the associated high rates of unemployment in young age groups in general.

Social class distribution shows similar patterns, with Pakistani and Bangladeshi groups showing a more disadvantaged profile. Perhaps most striking is the number of people from all minority ethnic groups who are living in poverty, as defined by less than half the average income. Just under a third of white households have incomes below this level, compared to a third of Chinese, two-fifths of African Caribbean and Indian households and four-fifths of Pakistani and Bangladeshi households[66]. Minority ethnic groups are also much more likely to be reliant on Income Support[67]. Although the 1991 Census showed a worse socioeconomic profile amongst Irish people, a recent survey shows that there are differences within the Irish, with men born in the Republic of Ireland being more likely to be in social class V than any other group. Men born in Northern Ireland, however, were more likely to be in social class I than men born in England, and as likely to be in social class II[435]. Another recent survey found relatively high proportions of Irish people amongst those earning more than £30,000 or with a university degree. Thus there may be some polarisation within the Irish group to different parts of the socioeconomic spectrum.

About four fifths of Indian and Pakistani households are owner occupied, compared with about two-thirds of white households and half of African Caribbean, Bangladeshi and Chinese households. Overcrowding is relatively common in minority ethnic households – one in ten African Caribbean and Indian households, and more than one in three Pakistani and Bangladeshi households compared with roughly one in fifty white households. Housing quality also varies. About a third of Pakistani and Bangladeshi people live in households which lack a basic amenity, for example, exclusive use of an inside toilet[66,441].

Evidence

The contribution of socioeconomic inequalities to inequalities in health both within and between ethnic groups has been much debated over the last twenty years. In an examination of migrant mortality data from the 1970s, there was no socioeconomic gradient for those born on the Indian sub-continent, and an association between higher socioeconomic status and higher mortality for those born in the Caribbean. Differences in socioeconomic status did not account for differences in mortality between migrant groups[447]. However, analysis of more recent data (1991–93) on migrant mortality has shown a relationship between socioeconomic status and health for some migrant groups[439].

All cause mortality was higher in men from manual classes than those from non-manual classes for all migrant groups, except those from West or South Africa, where the difference was present but smaller. In general this pattern was similar for the major causes of death, with the exception of coronary heart disease in men born in the Caribbean. Similar gradients have been found for self-reported health in a recent survey of minority ethnic groups[441]. Thus within minority ethnic groups in Britain, lower socioeconomic status is associated with higher rates of both mortality and morbidity.

However, it is not clear to what extent socioeconomic status accounts for differences in health between ethnic groups. The most recent analysis of migrant mortality suggests that socioeconomic differences, as measured by social class, do not explain

the different rates of mortality between groups born in different countries[439].
However coding of socioeconomic status using occupation, as in social class, may be a
particularly inappropriate proxy in migrants because of the high proportion of young
people and women amongst them who have never worked. Within any band of social
class, minority ethnic groups tend to be less advantaged than the majority white
population. For example, mean income for Pakistanis and Bangladeshis is about half
that found for whites in the same social class category[441].

The Fourth National Survey of Ethnic Minorities used an alternative index, standard of
living, which took into account material deprivation, measured by housing problems,
and ownership of cars and consumer durables. Socioeconomic status as measured by
this index did account for some of the differences in reported health between most
ethnic groups, whilst occupational class did not[441]. Thus socioeconomic inequalities
contribute to the inequalities in health within ethnic groups, and may contribute to
the inequalities in health between ethnic groups.

The diversity of experience of health between different ethnic groups may reflect
different causes of poor health; differential susceptibility to these causes; differential
access to factors which ameliorate cause or susceptibility, for example, preventive
health care services; or a combination of these. The Inquiry has decided to make
recommendations in two general areas. Firstly, there are recommendations aimed at
reducing the inequalities across ethnic groups in the socioeconomic determinants of
health, given the clear evidence that these are important determinants of health in
people from minority ethnic groups as they are for the ethnic majority. Secondly, there
are recommendations addressed at considering the needs of people from minority
ethnic groups in using services, particularly health services, which will ameliorate
their experience of ill-health.

The main examples of recommendations to address differences in health across
ethnic groups are considered here with a summary of their relevance to inequalities
across ethnic groups, in addition to their earlier consideration in appropriate parts of
the preceding text. Other recommendations may have relevance to inequalities across
ethnic groups to some degree.

Benefit

In general, the benefits from policies considered here would be expected to decrease
inequalities in health within ethnic groups. The benefit of such policies should be
relatively wide, and be felt by those within each group who are least well off. Because
minority ethnic communities typically contain a higher proportion of households with
children than the white population, these communities should benefit from policies
targeted at mothers, children and families (recommendations 2 and 21–23) and those
related to education (recommendation 4–7). The extent to which such policies will
decrease differences between ethnic groups is unknown. But the balance of evidence
would favour a reduction in inequalities between groups.

Considering the needs of people in different minority ethnic groups

Although separate mechanisms might be set up to consider policies which affect inequalities in health amongst minority ethnic groups, this risks marginalising minority ethnic issues. It also implies that the health problems in minority ethnic groups are, in the main, different from those in the ethnic majority, with different causes and different solutions, whereas in fact the similarities are greater than the differences[448,449]. However, failure to make specific consideration of minority ethnic issues risks increasing ethnic inequalities by unintentionally favouring policies that benefit the ethnic majority. Thus policies to consider inequalities in health should include consideration of the application of these policies to minority ethnic groups as a matter of course, including ways of ensuring that racial prejudice and harassment are overcome. This requires that the structures and processes of policy-making are sensitive to the position and needs of people from minority ethnic groups. One way of achieving this is to ensure that minority ethnic groups are represented on appropriate decision-making and advisory bodies, and that other opportunities are taken to seek their views. As well as the direct effect of such representation, the visibility of people from minority ethnic groups in such positions may reduce the sense of exclusion felt by some group members.

31. We RECOMMEND that the needs of minority ethnic groups are specifically considered in the development and implementation of policies aimed at reducing socioeconomic inequalities.

Reducing poverty

People from minority ethnic groups have higher than average rates of unemployment[40,45]. Within minority ethnic groups, there is a clear association between material disadvantage and poor health. Very high proportions of people from some minority ethnic groups are living on low levels of income, and are dependent on state benefits. There are a number of ways in which members of minority ethnic groups may be disadvantaged by the social security system. Some of the potential problems are related to the structure of the system and its assumptions. The State pension, for example, is based increasingly on the assumption that retired people should have built up occupational or other personal provisions over their working lives, but this would be impossible for people who migrated to Britain well into their working lives. Other problems are due to a failure to consider the specific needs of members of minority ethnic groups, for instance for translated or additional information[450-452]. Lack of these may lead to under-claiming of benefits. The younger demographic structure of many minority ethnic groups means that policies which improve the welfare of women of childbearing age, expectant mothers and children are of particular importance.

We recommend policies which will further reduce income inequalities, and improve the living standards of households in receipt of social security benefits (recommendation 3).

We recommend policies which improve the opportunities for work and which ameliorate the health consequences of unemployment (recommendation 8).

Improving housing, safety and the material environment

Although owner occupation is quite high in some minority ethnic groups, housing quality is often poor, regardless of tenure[441]. Overcrowding and lack of basic amenities is more common in some minority ethnic groups. Furthermore, current housing policy supports construction of homes for relatively small households, whereas for some minority ethnic groups, including Bangladeshis and Pakistanis, requests for housing are to accommodate extended family households. In addition, some minority ethnic groups find that their choice of area of residence is restricted by fear of crime and harassment[453].

We recommend policies which improve the availability of social housing for the less well off within a framework of environmental improvement, planning and design which takes into account social networks, and access to goods and services (recommendation 10).

We recommend policies which aim to improve the quality of housing (recommendation 12).

Responses to the Fourth National Survey on Ethnic Minorities suggested that more than one in eight people from minority ethnic groups had experienced some form of racial harassment in the past year[66]. Although most of these comprised racial insults, many respondents reported repeated victimisation and a quarter of all respondents reported being fearful of racial harassment. The British Crime Surveys have shown that South Asians and African Caribbeans are at greater risk of being victims of crime than whites. Although much of the difference in relation to African Caribbeans was explained by social and demographic factors, these did not explain the greater risk of victimisation for South Asians[222].

We recommend the development of policies to reduce the fear of crime and violence, and to create a safe environment for people to live in (recommendation 13).

The use and effects of transport on ethnic minorities has been little researched, partly because of a lack of relevant data[454,455]. Areas, particularly inner urban areas, with high proportions of minority ethnic residents are often characterised by markers of disadvantage[434,436]. These include on-street parking, higher traffic volumes and lack of areas for play, and are associated with a high rate of traffic accidents amongst children from some minority ethnic groups[456].

We recommend the further development of a high quality public transport system which is integrated with other forms of transport and is affordable to the user (recommendation 14).

We recommend further measures to encourage walking and cycling as forms of transport and to ensure the safe separation of pedestrians and cyclists from motor vehicles (recommendation 15).

We recommend further steps to reduce the usage of motor cars to cut the mortality and morbidity associated with motor vehicle emissions (recommendation 16).

We recommend further measures to reduce traffic speed, by environmental design and modification of roads, lower speed limits in built up areas, and stricter enforcement of speed limits (recommendation 17).

We recommend concessionary fares should be available to pensioners and disadvantaged groups throughout the country, and that local schemes should emulate high quality schemes, such as those of London and the West Midlands (recommendation 18).

Improving services

A number of studies have suggested that people from minority ethnic groups do not receive the same quality of care as the ethnic majority. Overall use of primary care is similar or greater amongst minority ethnic groups to the ethnic majority but people from minority ethnic groups are more likely than whites to: find physical access to their general practitioner (GP) difficult; have longer waiting times in the surgery; feel that the time spent with them was inadequate; and be less satisfied with the outcome of the consultation[441,457]. They may also be less likely to be referred to secondary and tertiary care[441,458-460]. Part of these differences may be related to problems with communication. A significant number of people from minority ethnic groups, particularly South Asian women and Chinese people, find it difficult to communicate with their GP[441,457]. There may also be cultural differences in the expression of symptoms, making the use of Western diagnostic approaches inappropriate for some groups, especially for mental illness[461]. Women from some minority ethnic groups, notably Pakistanis and Bangladeshis, prefer to consult with female doctors and in order to overcome communication difficulties, female doctors with the same minority ethnic background as themselves[441]. Given the younger demographic structure of many minority ethnic groups, the provision of sensitive maternal and child health services is of particular importance.

An illustrative example is ethnic differences in cervical screening. A national survey carried out recently found that South Asian women, especially Pakistani and Bangladeshi women, were less likely to have had a cervical smear in the past five years. About half of the Pakistani and Bangladeshi non-attenders lacked basic information about cervical screening, that is reported that they had not received an appointment or did not know what the test was[457]. Yet in a qualitative study carried out in the same period in East London, women from minority ethnic groups were enthusiastic about cervical cytology screening once they understood the purpose of the test and its procedures. Administrative and language barriers were important factors in participation in the screening programme, as were the adequacy of surgery premises[462].

One solution is to train health workers in "cultural competency". This involves acquiring the skills to understand and be sensitive to cultural differences in the presentation of illness and treatment, and other dimensions of health[463]. Bilingual link workers can act as translators and advocates for people from minority ethnic groups who experience communication problems with health care professionals. Support for health professionals such as general practitioners and health visitors who are themselves from minority ethnic groups is a further strategy to increase the quality of services to people from minority ethnic groups.

People from minority ethnic groups tend to congregate in specific geographical locations, which are frequently areas of multiple disadvantage[434,436]. Place as well as individual disadvantage may affect health[464,465]. However, the concentration of people from minority ethnic groups in particular areas may also be protective of health, by preserving levels of social support and a sense of community[466-468]. The advantages and disadvantages are likely to be conditional upon the place, and the minority ethnic group living there, making local consideration of policies to reduce inequalities essential.

32. We RECOMMEND *the further development of services which are sensitive to the needs of minority ethnic people and which promote greater awareness of their health risks.*

33. We RECOMMEND *the needs of minority ethnic groups are specifically considered in needs assessment, resource allocation, health care planning and provision.*

There are limitations on data currently collected to assess inequalities in health across ethnic groups. Death registration collects only country of birth, and so only mortality of migrants can be considered. Yet almost half of those who identified themselves as belonging to a minority ethnic group on Census night in 1991 had been born in the United Kingdom. The high proportions of young people and women who have never held a job, and the downward social mobility that may accompany immigration, mean that classification based on occupation is inappropriate as a measure of socioeconomic status in minority ethnic groups, particularly in comparison to the ethnic majority[441]. Grouping of minority ethnic people, such as Black or South Asian, may be inappropriate, merging together people who have different cultures, religion, migration history, socioeconomic status and geographical location.

We recommend a review of data needs to improve the capacity to monitor inequalities in health and their determinants at a national and local level (recommendation 1.2).

11. Gender

Introduction

Gender, like socioeconomic status, shapes individual opportunities and experiences across the life course. While many experiences of childhood are similar for boys and girls, they are exposed to different risks. Men and women occupy different positions in the labour market and in the home, which again bring different health risks.

Inequality

Mortality and life expectancy

Mortality is greater in males at all ages. In childhood, from 1 to 14 years, the higher mortality rates in boys are because they are more likely to die from poisoning and injury, including motor vehicle accidents, fire and flames, accidental drowning and submersion. The gender difference in mortality rates widens in the teenage years so that by the age of 15 years boys have 65 per cent higher mortality than girls. Over the last 20 years, the difference in childhood mortality rates between boys and girls has remained constant, despite falls in overall mortality[62].

In adult life, mortality is also greater in men. This is most pronounced in youth and early adulthood. For instance, the mortality rate is 2.8 times higher for men than for women aged 20–24 years. In youth and early adult life, the cause of the differences in mortality rates is the higher rates of male death from motor vehicle accidents, other accidents and suicide. Furthermore, mortality rates for women aged 25–40 have declined over the last 20 years, whereas those for men of the same age have increased[469,470].

Across the whole of adult life, mortality rates are higher for men than women for all the major causes of death. These include cancers and cardiovascular disease. However, the specific cancers vary between the sexes. In women, breast cancer is the most common neoplasm to cause death (lung cancer is the second most common), whereas in men it is lung cancer (prostate cancer is the second most common). The overall fall in mortality rates since 1971 has been accompanied by a slight reduction in the differential death rates between men and women. In 1971 males had a 64 per cent higher mortality rate than women. By 1996 this had reduced to a 55 per cent higher rate in men[25].

Life expectancy is 5 years longer in women than in men. Overall life expectancy has increased for both sexes throughout this century[26]. Recently, the increases have been slightly greater for men than women, reversing an earlier slight trend in the opposite direction. However, for healthy life expectancy, that is years of life free of disability or chronic illness, there is a smaller gender difference. Women have a 2 to 3 year greater expectancy of healthy life than men. Overall healthy life expectancy has changed little over the last 10 years and the difference between men and women has also remained constant[27].

The choice of measure of socioeconomic status may influence the pattern of health inequalities observed. For example, measures based on occupation may reflect different facets of life for men compared to women, but the extent to which this affects observed patterns of health between and within sexes is unknown. Using the Townsend index as a measure of deprivation, the different effects of socioeconomic status and gender are such that the least well off women still have lower mortality rates than the most well off men (figure 16)[73]. In general, gender differences in mortality are smaller in areas of relative affluence and greater in the most economically deprived areas[471,472].

Furthermore, there are differences between the genders in the magnitude of the socioeconomic gradient in mortality. Analyses have shown that, for all-cause mortality, the gradient is steeper in men than in women, and that this is also the case for the major causes of death, with the exception of cardiovascular disease[471,472]. These differences between and within genders have important policy implications.

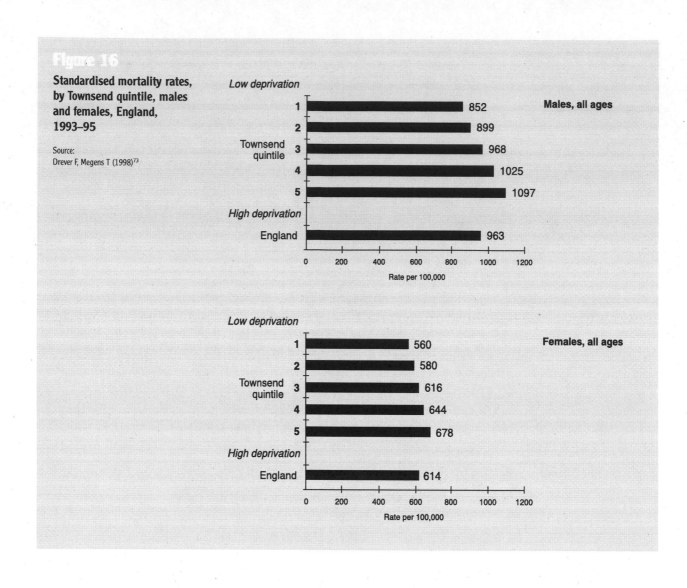

Figure 16

Standardised mortality rates, by Townsend quintile, males and females, England, 1993–95

Source:
Drever F, Megens T (1998)[73]

Males, all ages

Townsend quintile	Rate per 100,000
1	852
2	899
3	968
4	1025
5	1097
England	963

Females, all ages

Townsend quintile	Rate per 100,000
1	560
2	580
3	616
4	644
5	678
England	614

They suggest that policies which decrease socioeconomic inequalities will have a differential effect by decreasing male mortality, and particularly mortality in more disadvantaged men. They also suggest the need for gender specific policies to reduce inequalities, because the causes of inequalities may be different for men and women.

Morbidity

A traditional view of gender differences in morbidity has been to highlight an apparent paradox: that males have higher mortality rates but females have higher rates of morbidity[473,474]. However, in more detailed analysis, this generalisation often does not hold true. For example, in adults, gender differences in global measures of health and well-being are relatively modest[475]. In people over 60 years of age, for instance, the difference in proportions of men and women in 5 year age bands who reported that they were in good health seldom varied by more than 5 per cent[474]. Furthermore, broad assumptions that females experience more ill-health than males conceal specific gender differences in both directions.

For children, boys are more likely to report long standing illness, 18 per cent for boys and 15 per cent for girls, although the difference is only 1 per cent greater in boys for limiting long standing illness. Boys are 30 to 40 per cent more likely than girls to have consulted at a general practice for serious conditions, but about 10 per cent less likely to have done so for minor conditions. Hospital admissions are higher for boys, although the difference from rates for girls has decreased somewhat[28]. A review of the interaction of gender and age during childhood concluded that while boys had higher rates of chronic physical illness in childhood, this pattern was reversed in early to mid-adolescence, when there were higher rates for girls. This pattern was repeated for psychological disorders, mostly neurotic, where an excess in young boys was replaced by an excess in girls by mid-adolescence[476]. One possibility is that the increased levels of physical complaints in adolescent girls arise, at least in part, as a result of the lowering of their psychological well-being at this age[476].

Women have more morbidity from poor mental health, particularly those related to anxiety and depressive disorders[38]. Furthermore, psychosocial health in women is strongly influenced by socioeconomic status. For example, a recent analysis of the socioeconomic patterning of women's health found that psychosocial well-being displayed the steepest socioeconomic gradient. Lone mothers had particularly poor psychosocial health, even after controlling for household income, employment status and occupation[477]. On the other hand, men have higher rates of alcohol and drug dependence[38].

Osteoporosis deserves special mention as it is a disabling condition which is more common in women. The lifetime risk from the age of 50 years of fracture of the hip, spine or distal forearm – for which osteoporosis is a major determinant – is 14 per cent, 11 per cent and 13 per cent respectively for women compared to 3 per cent, 2 per cent and 2 per cent for men. The causes of the differences in fracture rates between men and women are not fully understood, but differences in bone density, size and architecture, together with a gender difference in falling, are likely to be major contributors[478].

Women have much higher rates of disability than men, especially at older ages[479]. Data from the 1994 General Household Survey showed that older women were more likely to experience restrictions of mobility, self-care and ability to perform household tasks than older men[480]. For instance, under a fifth of men over the age of 85 years were unable to go out and walk down the road, compared with nearly half of women. When measures of functional impairment are combined – ability to get up and down stairs, walking outside, getting around the house, ability to bathe or wash oneself, to cut toenails and to get in and out of bed – 14 per cent of women over the age of 65 years suffer from functional impairments sufficient to require help on a daily basis to remain living in the community, compared to only 7 per cent of men. By the age of 85 and over, these figures have risen to nearly 40 per cent for women and 21 per cent for men[474]. As a consequence, the 1991 Census showed that twice as many women as men over the age of 65 years lived in a communal establishment, 6.4 per cent of women compared to 3 per cent of men[481].

Health related behaviour

The proportion of both men and women who smoke has decreased over the last 20 years, but this decrease has been proportionately more in men so that there is now no differential in rates between men and women smoking. About 6 to 7 per cent of men drink alcohol very heavily, based on the (now discontinued) definition of more than 50 units per week. This compares to 2 per cent of women, drinking more than 35 units per week. These proportions, and the proportions who drink heavily, have changed little over the past 10 years. Women are more likely than men to eat wholemeal bread, fruit and vegetables at least once per day, and to drink semi-skimmed milk[35]. They are also more likely to diet[270]. Levels of physical activity are higher in men than women, but this is mainly due to men's higher levels of occupational activity[35].

In children and adolescents, the patterns are slightly different, and may herald differences in future gender patterns of adult health related behaviour. Secondary school-aged girls have higher rates of regular smoking than boys, although boys who are regular smokers smoke more tobacco[63]. Higher smoking prevalence among girls has been reported since regular national surveys of school children were first conducted in 1982. If these gender differences were carried forward into adulthood, there should now be evidence of higher rates of smoking among women than men in the 16–24 age group, and to a lesser extent, in the 25–34 age group. Since these trends are not in evidence, it appears that the gender difference in smoking observed among school children is transient[482]. Boys tend to drink alcohol more often than girls and to consume more when they do drink[63]. But girls are more likely to have been offered illegal drugs[117]. Girls tend to eat fruit and vegetables more often than boys, but also eat more less "healthy" foods, such as cakes and chips, and tend to go without breakfast. By year 11 of secondary school, 23 per cent of girls are dieting and only about half are happy with their weight[117]. Girls spend less of their free time playing games or sport[483,484].

Socioeconomic determinants

There are important gender differences in factors which are associated with health, and which the Inquiry has taken the view are determinants of health. Despite women's increased participation in paid employment over the past 30 years, women and men occupy very different positions in and outside the labour market. Nearly 30 per cent of women of working age are economically inactive, and only 35 per cent work full-time; among men, 16 per cent are economically inactive and nearly 60 per cent work full-time[42]. Over half the female labour force is employed in the clerical, personal and retail sectors as secretaries, waitresses, hairdressers, checkout operators etc., sectors characterised by low paid work[485,486]. Among men, less than one fifth work in these services[485]. Outside the labour market, it is women rather than men who take primary responsibility for keeping the home and family going: doing the shopping, cooking and housework and caring for children and other relatives[487]. Forty per cent of women spend over 50 hours a week caring for someone living with them[488].

Gender differences in educational qualifications vary by age and measure. In 1997, 23 per cent of women of working age had no qualifications compared with 16 per cent of men[45]. By contrast girls are more likely to gain 5 or more GCSEs at grades A star to C than boys[41].

Women's different positions in the labour market and in the home means that they live more home-based and community-based lives, where they provide for the health needs of vulnerable groups, including children and adults with long term needs for care. Their different occupational and domestic positions also make women more vulnerable to poverty than men, both during their reproductive and working lives and in old age. It has been estimated that two thirds of adults in the poorest households are women, and women make up 60 per cent of adults in households dependent on Income Support[76]. Because women are more likely to have breaks in employment and to work part-time in low paying jobs, they are less likely to be eligible for and in receipt of contributory benefits than men and more likely to be on means-tested benefits, both before and after retirement age[77,489]. Among those aged 65 or over, for example, there are three times as many female as male recipients of Income Support[77]. Social isolation is also more likely in women than men. Women are less likely to be able to drive or to have access to a car[40,282]. Older women are more likely than older men to be widowed and to live alone[420,421].

In summary, despite their more favourable position with respect to socioeconomic determinants of health, males have higher mortality rates. Gender differences in morbidity vary according to the age group under consideration, the type of morbidity being measured and the measure used.

Evidence

The Inquiry has considered the evidence on gender inequalities in three ways. Firstly, there are obvious differences in the health of males and females which relate to their different biology. Such differences include, for instance, the differences between the sexes in specific diseases of the reproductive organs, and the ill health that may be associated with childbearing. The Inquiry has sought to identify determinants of or solutions to gender-specific health states which are amenable to policy intervention. An example is policies to prevent unwanted teenage pregnancy. Unwanted teenage pregnancy is more common in girls from disadvantaged backgrounds and is associated with a range of adverse health outcomes. Gender inequalities of this type have been considered at appropriate points in the preceding text and are not considered again in this section.

Secondly, there are gender differences in health that do not appear to be predicated on inevitable differences in biology. An example is the higher rate of accidental death in young adult males. Accidental death is associated with lower socioeconomic status, yet low socioeconomic status (as measured by employment status) is more common amongst young women than young men[490]. This suggests that the gender difference in death rates from accidents reflects social and cultural influences which have a differential impact on men and women. These types of inequalities are likely to be amenable to policy interventions. They have been considered in the appropriate sections of the preceding text and the main examples are re-considered in this section with a summary of their relevance to gender differences. Other recommendations may also have some relevance to gender inequalities.

Thirdly, there are differences between genders in wider aspects of health, particularly mental and social health. An example is the existence of food poverty amongst lone mothers living on state benefits[93,94]. This is likely to be less common amongst men of the same age because they are less likely to be living in these circumstances. Going without food because of lack of money might not be within the definition of morbidity but it can hardly be described as a healthy state. Similarly, cultural expectations of male and female roles may mean that the frustrations, hopelessness and loss of self-esteem associated with unemployment are felt more keenly by the male partner of an unemployed couple, even if both are seeking work. Again, such feelings are not compatible with good mental health, although they would not be described as psychiatric morbidity. In addition to their earlier consideration in appropriate parts of the preceding text, the main examples of recommendations to address gender differences in these wider aspects of health are considered specifically here, with a summary of their relevance to gender inequalities. Again, other recommendations, not reconsidered here, may have relevance to such gender inequalities to some degree.

We have focused our recommendations in three areas: reducing death in young men; improving health is disadvantaged women with young children; and reducing disability in older women.

Benefit

In general, the benefits from policies considered here will decrease gender inequalities by decreasing disadvantage to either males or females. The benefit of such policies should therefore be relatively wide, and be felt by those males or females who are least well off. However, the mechanisms which link social and cultural influences to differences in male and female health are not well understood. Partly as a consequence, the differential effect on male and female health of policies is often unknown.

Finally, it should be noted that policies which improve the health of women of childbearing age may, in addition, improve the health of the next generation[21]. This may itself have implications for gender differences in health, as males may be more susceptible to some adverse events in utero and early life than females[21]. For example, boys are more susceptible than girls to the long term effects of postnatal depression in their mothers[342].

Reducing death in young men

Our policies in this area aim to reduce deaths from accidents and suicide. Mortality from road traffic accidents is higher in males of all ages[25]. The policies which we recommend may have a differential effect on males, particularly those in lower socioeconomic groups, because they are aimed at reducing the opportunity for, or enforcing limits on, risk-taking behaviour as a pedestrian or motor vehicle user.

In England and Wales in 1996, the age-standardised mortality rate for suicide was three times higher in males than in females – 137 and 44 per million respectively[29]. The overall rate has fallen by nearly a half in women over the last 20 years, but there has been little change in men. For men under the age of 44 years, however, there has been a rise of 20–30 per cent, compared to a fall of about the same magnitude in men over this age[32]. There is a steep social class gradient in deaths from suicide. In 1991–1993, rates for men were 4 times higher in social class V than in social class I. Our policies aim to reduce the causes of social exclusion which lead to despair and to improve mental health services for people who are already mentally ill. Detailed evidence in support of these recommendations is given at appropriate points in the preceding text.

34. We RECOMMEND policies which reduce the excess mortality from accidents and suicide in young men. Specifically:

we recommend policies which improve the opportunities for work and which ameliorate the health consequences of unemployment (recommendation 8).

We recommend policies which improve housing provision and access to health care for both officially and unofficially homeless people (recommendation 11).

We recommend further measures to encourage walking and cycling as forms of transport and to ensure the safe separation of pedestrians and cyclists from motor vehicles (recommendation 15).

We recommend further steps to reduce the usage of motor cars to cut the mortality and morbidity associated with motor vehicle emissions (recommendation 16).

We recommend further measures to reduce traffic speed, by environmental design and modification of roads, lower speed limits in built up areas, and stricter enforcement of speed limits (recommendation 17).

We recommend policies to prevent suicide among young people, especially among young men and seriously mentally ill people (recommendation 24).

We recommend policies which reduce alcohol-related ill health, accidents and violence, including measures which at least maintain the real cost of alcohol (recommendation 26.5).

Improving health in disadvantaged women with young children

Women are more likely than men to take primary responsibility for caring for children and other relatives[487]. Forty per cent of women spend over 50 hours per week caring for someone living with them[488]. Improving the conditions – financial, social and environmental – in which women in poorer circumstances care for their families is likely to be an essential part of any strategy to reduce socioeconomic inequalities in health. People on low incomes or reliant on state benefits are more likely to be lone parents, most of whom are women[65]. Furthermore, current levels of benefit fall short of the level which independent experts determine to be the modern minimum[78,80,81,84,85]. Lone mothers may go without food because of lack of money, and some have nutritionally deficient diets[93–95,116].

Caring for young children in disadvantaged circumstances, particularly as a lone mother, carries with it an increased risk of poor mental health. In the Health and Lifestyle Survey, the most important factor associated with the mental health of married women aged under 45 years, was the age of their youngest child. Women with children under the age of 5 were most likely to show signs of psychological disturbance. The age of youngest child had no association with physical health[491]. In a survey of 11,000 mothers 8 months after birth (the Avon Longitudinal Study of Pregnancy and Childhood), material disadvantage was more strongly related to stress-related conditions such as depression, anxiety and headache/migraine, than to conditions like backache, haemorrhoids and cough/cold. For the former conditions, higher levels of self-reported morbidity and general practitioner consultation were associated with a cluster of social disadvantages – living in rented housing, non-employment, younger age, lower educational status. Having more than one child was associated with higher self-reported morbidity for both depression and anxiety[492].

Women of all ages are more likely than men to be reliant on public transport, especially buses. Fewer women than men can drive, and fewer women than men own or have access to a car[40,282]. Surveys in a number of UK cities have found that around two thirds of women are afraid to go out alone at night, and that significant numbers will not use public transport because of fears for personal safety[493]. This combination of lack of access to transport and fear for safety is likely to decrease opportunities for access to family and friends, facilities and services.

Policies aimed at the material, social and emotional support of women who are pregnant or who have young children should lead to improved psychosocial health in the mother and related improvements in the health of their children. These improvements should be felt in many aspects of health and its determinants, and be apparent in the short and long term. Detailed evidence in support of these recommendations is given at the appropriate points in the preceding text.

35. We RECOMMEND policies which reduce psychosocial ill health in young women in disadvantaged circumstances, particularly those caring for young children. Specifically:

we recommend further reductions in poverty in women of childbearing age, expectant mothers, young children and older people should be made by increasing benefits in cash or in kind to them (recommendation 3.1).

We recommend uprating of benefits and pensions according to principles which protect and, where possible, improve the standard of living of those who depend on them, and which narrow the gap between their standard of living and average living standards (recommendation 3.2).

We recommend measures to increase the uptake of benefits in entitled groups (recommendation 3.3).

We recommend policies which improve the availability of social housing for the less well off within a framework of environmental improvement, planning and design which takes into account social networks, and access to goods and services (recommendation 10).

We recommend the further development of a high quality public transport system which is integrated with other forms of transport and is affordable to the user (recommendation 14).

We recommend policies which will increase the availability and accessibility of foodstuffs to supply an adequate and affordable diet (recommendation 20).

We recommend policies which reduce poverty in families with children by promoting the material support of parents; by removing barriers to work for parents who wish to combine work with parenting; and enabling those who wish to devote full-time to parenting to do so (recommendation 21).

We recommend an integrated policy for the provision of affordable, high quality day care and pre-school education with extra resources for disadvantaged communities (recommendation 21.1).

We recommend policies which improve the health and nutrition of women of childbearing age and their children with priority given to the elimination of food poverty and the prevention and reduction of obesity (recommendation 22).

We recommend policies which promote the social and emotional support for parents and children (recommendation 23).

We recommend the further development of the role and capacity of health visitors to provide social and emotional support to expectant parents, and parents with young children (recommendation 23.1).

We recommend policies which promote sexual health in young people and reduce unwanted teenage pregnancy, including access to appropriate contraceptive services (recommendation 25).

Reducing disability in older women

People on low incomes or reliant on state benefits are more likely to be lone parents, especially women, or pensioners, the majority of whom are women. Only a quarter of older women have an occupational or personal pension compared to two thirds of older men[494]. Low income decreases their chances of maintaining autonomy and independence by rendering them unable to pay for transport, social care and aids or adaptations to compensate for functional disability[474].

Properties in poor condition are occupied disproportionately by single older people, the majority of whom are women[209]. These homes have higher heating costs. The combination of living alone, and on a low income, puts older women at high risk of fuel poverty[96,97,474].

Women of all ages are more likely than men to be reliant on public transport, especially buses. Fewer women than men can drive, and fewer women than men own or have access to a car. This gender difference is most pronounced for older women[40,282]. Surveys in a number of UK cities have found that around two thirds of women are afraid to go out alone at night, and that significant numbers will not use public transport because of fears for personal safety[220,493]. Fear for personal safety is greater in older women than those of younger ages. Older women are more likely to live alone than older men[420,421], and thus need to go out in order to access social networks.

Older women are more likely than older men to suffer from functional impairments sufficient to require help on a daily basis to remain living in the community[474]. Changes in community care policies in the early 1990s made it more difficult for older people to obtain local authority residential or home care. Such policies have had a greater effect on older women. Older men are more likely than older women to have the financial resources to pay for such care, and are more likely to be living with a wife, who can contribute to care[420,421]. Older disabled women are twice as likely as men with a comparable level of disability to live alone[474].

Our recommendations are aimed at the reduction of disability in older women, by improving the material support to them, the environment in which they live, and access to the services which they need. Detailed evidence in support of these recommendations is given at appropriate points in the preceding text.

36. We RECOMMEND policies which reduce disability and ameliorate its consequences in older women, particularly those living alone. Specifically:

we recommend further reductions in poverty in women of childbearing age, expectant mothers, young children and older people should be made by increasing benefits in cash or in kind to them (recommendation 3.1).

We recommend uprating of benefits and pensions according to principles which protect and, where possible, improve the standard of living of those who depend on them and which narrow the gap between their standard of living and average living standards (recommendation 3.2).

We recommend measures to increase the uptake of benefits in entitled groups (recommendation 3.3).

We recommend the development of policies to reduce the fear of crime and violence, and to create a safe environment for people to live in (recommendation 13).

We recommend the further development of a high quality public transport system which is integrated with other forms of transport and is affordable to the user (recommendation 14).

We recommend concessionary fares should be available to pensioners and disadvantaged groups throughout the country, and that local schemes should emulate high quality schemes, such as those of London and the West Midlands (recommendation 18).

We recommend the quality of homes in which older people live be improved (recommendation 28).

We recommend the further development of health and social services for older people, so that these services are accessible and distributed according to need (recommendation 30).

The National Health Service

The institutional links to Government, whereby the Secretary of State for Health is responsible for the service, gives the National Health Service (NHS) a different status from the areas for policy development considered earlier in the report. For this reason, we have set out this section and our recommendations slightly differently, focusing on management and operational issues. However, as for the rest of the report, we have based our recommendations on scientific and expert evidence.

Equity

Equity was a founding principle of the NHS[495] and is central to Government policy[5,87].

The NHS has several interlinked responsibilities in relation to health inequalities:
- to provide equity of access to effective health care
- to work in partnership with other agencies to improve health and tackle the causes of health inequalities
- to provide professional leadership and to stimulate the development of health policies beyond the boundaries of the NHS[13,14].

This chapter examines what is known about the relationship of socioeconomic variations in health to equity in health care and what action could be taken by the NHS in conjunction with others to reduce health inequalities.

The principle of equity includes several important elements: ensuring that health care services serving disadvantaged populations are not of poorer quality or less accessible; that the allocation and application of resources are in relation to need; and ensuring that positive efforts are made to achieve greater uptake and use of effective services by making extra efforts to reach those whose health is worse.

Equity in access to health care

Differences in access to preventive health care or treatment services do not necessarily indicate inequity in access between social groups unless these differences are adjusted for need. A recent systematic review indicated that much of the research on inequities in access to health care neither adjusted for need nor for socioeconomic factors[496]. Furthermore relatively little research has studied the effects of variations in health care treatments on the course of disease and the reasons for differential survival between social groups.

We have considered inequalities in relation to primary care, secondary care, including specialist care, and mental health services. Our overriding perspective has been that the NHS, should, above all, be aiming to provide equitable access to effective health care for those who need it. In the case of primary care, it is important that services are readily accessible as well as effective. For some specialist hospital services, a different balance needs to be struck between local access and securing an effective critical mass of services to achieve the best outcomes[497].

Inequities in access to primary care

Access to effective primary care is influenced by several "supply" factors: the geographical distribution and availability of primary care staff, the range and quality of primary care facilities, levels of training, education and recruitment of primary care staff, cultural sensitivity, timing and organisation of services to the communities served, distance, and the availability of affordable and safe means of transport. "Demand" factors such as lay health beliefs, knowing what services are available locally and wider socioeconomic influences, such as financial insecurity, social mobility and lack of informal carer support will also affect patterns of utilisation and access to health care.

Higher rates of general practitioner (GP) consultation are associated with greater social and economic deprivation even after adjusting for need[496]. However, the further away patients live from their GP, the less frequently they tend to consult. This is evident in rural areas – although the differences are not as great for serious health problems as for less severe ones[498].

Communities most at risk of ill health tend to experience the least satisfactory access to the full range of preventive services, the so called "inverse prevention law". Prevention services include cancer screening programmes, health promotion and immunisation. While differences are most noticeable amongst socioeconomic groups it is likely that, for example amongst Bangladeshi women, additional inequalities in access are experienced[499]. Lack of access to women practitioners can be a deterrent to Asian women taking up an invitation for cervical cancer screening[462]. Local studies have shown that access to female practitioners is poorest in areas with high concentrations of Asian residents[500] and that practices with a female doctor or nurse are more likely to reach the cervical cytology targets set out in the GP contract[501]. Sub-regional and small area analyses illustrate this inequity for areas such as Liverpool[502] and Birmingham where, using nine indicators of primary care services, the most deprived areas tended to be the least well served[500]. Within London, health promotion claims by GPs are highest in the least deprived and lowest in the most deprived areas (figure 17)[503].

Inequities in access to secondary care

Evidence on variations in access to secondary care is often difficult to interpret, since many studies do not adjust for case mix or distinguish between emergency and

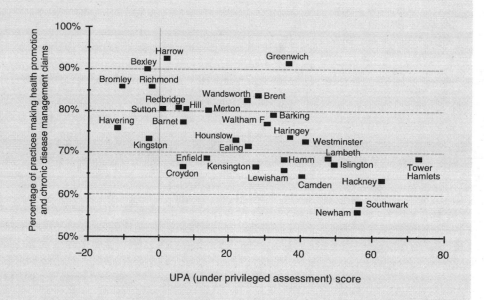

Figure 17

GP health promotion claims, by Jarman (UPA) score of health authority, London Boroughs, October 1995

Source:
Bardsley M, *et al.* (1997)[503]

elective care. Monitoring equity of access to secondary care from routine data sources is also difficult, since the collection of data about ethnicity, socioeconomic status and utilisation of the private sector is incomplete.

There is a positive relationship between levels of deprivation in an area and hospital admission rates, although there are great variations in hospital admission rates between GP practices[504,505]. Thus deprivation is not the only factor influencing hospital admission and higher admission rates could also in part reflect poorer access to primary and community care services, as for example in the case of diabetes and asthma[506].

For out-patients, attendance is either higher in disadvantaged groups or similar to the better off, after adjusting for need. For some minority ethnic groups out-patients attendance rates are lower than for the ethnic majority[496]. There is some evidence to suggest this may be related to GP referral beliefs and practices[458,507]. Inequity in access to investigation and specialist cardiac services treatment has been observed in relation to socioeconomic factors, ethnic group, gender, age and geography. For example, since mortality from coronary heart disease in South Asians is 40 per cent higher than the general population, intervention rates for large Asian communities might be expected to be higher than average. The evidence shows the opposite after adjusting for socioeconomic and geographical factors[496]. Similarly, rates for coronary artery bypass grafts and and coronary angioplasty are not generally higher in areas with the greatest need (figure 18)[508, 509]. For many other NHS hospital treatments, there is little evidence of systematic inequities in access between deprivation groups[509].

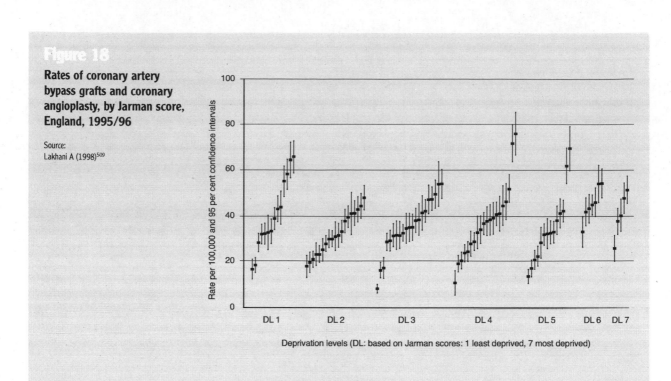

Figure 18

Rates of coronary artery bypass grafts and coronary angioplasty, by Jarman score, England, 1995/96

Source:
Lakhani A (1998)[509]

Deprivation levels (DL: based on Jarman scores: 1 least deprived, 7 most deprived)

Inequities in access to mental health services

Mental health services, although specialist in nature, are both community and hospital based. Here we focus on the link between social deprivation and serious mental illness and utilisation of mental health services. The use of psychiatric – especially inpatient hospital services – is positively correlated with high levels of deprivation and unemployment[496]. There is also evidence of high inpatient admission rates for schizophrenia but lower consultation rates for mental health problems among young African Caribbean men[496]. In contrast, women and men from South Asian populations have much lower rates of GP consultation for mental health problems than the white population[507,510].

There is a lack of consensus about the explanation for these different patterns of utilisation. Over-representation of young male African Caribbeans in the inpatient sector may be due to higher levels of need or, alternatively, racial discrimination within both the NHS and criminal justice systems. Equally, it is not clear whether the observed under-utilisation by Asians represents inequities in access to services or an appropriate response to lower levels of need. Whatever the explanation of these differences in access, it is clear that, given the high prevalence of severe mental illness in the local population, mental health services in inner cities have difficulty in coping with demand[511].

The allocation of resources for mental health services should be sufficiently weighted to meet the needs of culturally diverse populations and to enable strategies to be developed which provide culturally appropriate services, and strengthen further developments of community based services within the NHS, local authority, voluntary and community sector. Such strategies need to consider other influences on mental health, such as housing and employment.

Clinical governance

Routine information systems are needed to alert clinicians and managers to changing patterns of access and health outcomes. We welcome the Government's intention to produce, after a developmental period, and make public, comparative information on clinical outcomes. We suggest that the best way of encouraging effective clinical governance is to ensure that valid, robust and user-friendly data are provided. The commitment to develop National Service Frameworks should reinforce this by setting and monitoring minimum standards.

37. *We RECOMMEND that providing equitable access to effective care in relation to need should be a governing principle of all policies in the NHS. Priority should be given to the achievement of equity in the planning, implementation and delivery of services at every level of the NHS. Specifically:*

37.1. *we recommend extending the focus of clinical governance to give equal prominence to equity of access to effective health care.*

37.2 *We recommend extending the remit of the National Institute for Clinical Excellence to include equity of access to effective health care.*

37.3 *We recommend developing the National Service Frameworks to address inequities in access to effective primary care.*

37.4 *We recommend that performance management in relation to the national performance management framework is focused on achieving more equitable access, provision and targeting of effective services in relation to need in both primary and hospital sectors.*

Providing equitable access to effective care should also include a process of monitoring the quality of local partnerships for health and social care, and the involvement of local people in the provision of services.

37.5 *We recommend that the Department of Health and NHS Executive set out their responsibilities for furthering the principle of equity of access to effective health and social care, and that health authorities, working with Primary Care Groups and providers on local clinical governance, agree priorities and objectives for reducing inequities in access to effective care. These should form part of the Health Improvement Programme.*

Resource allocation

We welcome the progress that has been made in recent years in achieving a more equitable approach to allocating health service and related resources. However, the evidence suggests that more needs to be done[512,513].

Firstly, the methodology for estimating the size of underenumerated, mobile and homeless populations needs to be improved in the census and inter-censal years. This is a particular problem for the allocation of resources to Primary Care Group populations.

Secondly, there is insufficient recognition of ethnic and cultural needs in the funding arrangements, such as the costs of bilingual advocates/interpretation which have been shown to improve health outcome in disadvantaged ethnic groups[514]. An "Ethnic Diversity Levy" and allocating it in relation to size, diversity and need identified by health authorities may provide a more effective targeting and accountability mechanism.

Primary care

An "inverse care law" is still evident in relation to the distribution of medical and nursing staff in relation to need[515]. A number of studies have also shown that deprived areas suffer increasing difficulty in recruiting GPs[516]. This situation has been exacerbated – especially in inner London – by the poor quality of primary care premises, large numbers of single-handed GPs, GPs approaching retirement and practices without training status[517-519]. This inequity extends beyond that of GPs to other primary care staff including practice nurses, health visitors and district nurses[520].

A formulaic approach such as the allocation of GPs to health authority areas, such as operated by the Medical Practices Committee, is unlikely to be sufficient as a policy to deal with the growing shortage of GPs in deprived inner city areas. Equally, the GP deprivation payment system whereby GPs working in deprived areas receive additional payments, whilst well-intentioned, has neither been effective in attracting GPs to these areas, nor in increasing access to effective services for disadvantaged populations[516,521]. Innovative schemes, such as the introduction of salaried GPs, have been shown to help redress some of these inequities[522].

Hospital and community health services (HCHS)

Despite the efforts to achieve greater equity in the allocation of HCHS services, evidence suggests that a number of issues still need to be addressed[512,513]. One is the pace by which health authorities move towards their target resource allocations and the way in which those resources are then spent. In 1998/99, if the top 20 per cent of health authorities in England were able to move to their target allocation, this would involve a shift of over £198 million from those currently over target. Such shifts of resources are large and would need careful planning, but need to be achieved if HCHS resources are to be distributed equitably (figure 19)[523].

Health promotion

Aside from specific health promotion payments in primary care, and ring-fenced HIV/AIDS and substance misuse funding, there is no recognition of a capitation or

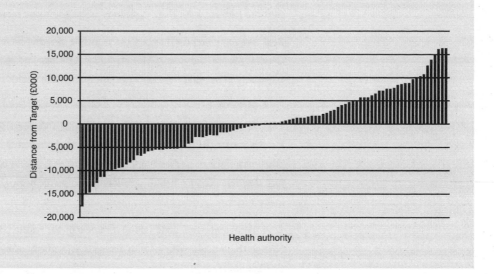

Figure 19

Distance from Resource Allocation Target, all health authorities, England, 1998/99

Source:
NHS Executive (1997)[523]

needs-based allocation to support health promotion services on a more comprehensive basis. The needs-based formula for targeting HIV prevention funds has achieved some success in allocating resources where they are most needed[524], although their use needs to be targeted and monitored more effectively. The principle of ring-fencing resources with greater accountability for their use could be used both visibly and effectively in local inter-agency work to support the principles of "Our Healthier Nation"[1].

The role of the private sector

The value of privately funded acute health care provided both within and independently of the NHS was estimated at £2.35 billion in 1996 with private revenue within the NHS estimated at £252 million in 1996/7[525].

A number of studies suggest that the distribution of, and access to, private health care compounds existing inequalities[526,527]. Currently, information on levels of activity and quality of private sector services is not routinely available. This means that no complete picture exists for both public and private sectors of access, resources and the outcomes of treatment in relation to need.

We suggest that those providing private health care should be required to give the same routine information on activity and quality of services as the NHS. This is already statutorily required in the case of assisted conceptions, abortions and nursing home care and such arrangements could be extended as part of the performance assessment framework. An independent review of private practice would enable full consideration of the relationship of private practice to the NHS, and its impact on equity issues.

38. We RECOMMEND giving priority to the achievement of a more equitable allocation of NHS resources. This will require adjustments to the ways in which resources are allocated and the speed with which resource allocation targets are met. Specifically:

38.1 we recommend reviewing the "pace of change" policy to enable health authorities that are furthest from their capitation targets to move more quickly to their actual target.

38.2 We recommend extending the principle of needs-based weighting to non-cash limited General Medical Services (GMS) resources. The size and effectiveness of deprivation payments in meeting the needs and improving the health outcomes amongst the most disadvantaged populations, including ethnic minorities should be assessed.

38.3 We recommend reviewing the size and effectiveness of the Hospital and Community Health Service (HCHS) formula and deprivation payments in influencing the health care outcomes of the most disadvantaged populations, and to consider alternative methods of focusing resources for health promotion and public health care to reduce health inequalities.

38.4 We recommend establishing a review of the relationship of private practice to the NHS with particular reference to access to effective treatments, resource allocation and availability of staff.

Local partnerships to reduce health inequalities

As many of the determinants of health inequalities lie outside the health care system, it is essential for the NHS to work effectively across organisational boundaries in partnership with local authorities, the voluntary and business sectors, to involve local people in developing and providing services, and to contribute actively to social and economic regeneration.

This shared responsibility for health is central to the idea of a local Health Improvement Programme, described in "Our Healthier Nation" and "The New NHS" White Paper[1,5], as well as such initiatives as Healthy Living Centres. These plans will need to be properly supported by appropriate mechanisms and underpinned by local commitment if they are to successfully play their part in a concerted national programme to improve health and tackle health inequalities[87].

Birmingham and Liverpool, cities whose health and local authorities are coterminous, have undertaken detailed analyses of inequalities within their boundaries[500,528]. Liverpool, the first to join the World Health Organisation's Healthy Cities initiative 10 years ago, has a joint City Health Plan based on a comprehensive review of health and its social, economic and educational determinants. More recently its employment, economic and regeneration strategies have been more closely aligned to health objectives. Whilst there is little evidence of any reduction in inequalities in most health areas, there is some evidence of a shift of primary care resources into areas of greatest need with a resultant increase in immunisation uptake[502]. A new index of quality of life and health has been developed to help monitor progress in implementing the plan.

Information about the supply of services and resources going into an area is not easy to obtain, but these types of "equity audit" are essential for developing a more strategic approach to addressing health and health care inequalities at a local level.

The NHS White Paper sets out five new vehicles for improving health and tackling health inequalities, as well as local Health Improvement Programmes[5]. They include Primary Care Groups, a new system of clinical governance, a duty of partnership between health and local authorities, and a new NHS performance assessment framework. The principle of equity needs to be given prominence as this framework is developed if inequalities in health are to be addressed in a co-ordinated way.

Developing the capacity for tackling health inequalities

In order to take forward a new agenda to tackle health inequalities, the skills, resources, and capacity of organisations to work together need to be strengthened. The Chief Medical Officer's interim report on strengthening the public health function identified the need for shared posts to support the creation of local health partnerships, work across organisational boundaries and involve local people in health promotion and service delivery[529]. One conclusion was that a well resourced multi-disciplinary network is required at each level of the health care system to take forward policy development, share innovation and good practice. Steps need to be taken nationally to ensure that the capacity for interagency working at local level is strengthened and that the resources and skills available for specialist health promotion, including professional and community development are protected.

National level

Health inequalities between social groups and between areas will not be reduced by local action alone. Local agencies will need the leadership and support of central Government and the European Union. This approach is relevant if new incentives and freedoms to working in partnership and sharing resources are to be created.

39. We RECOMMEND Directors of Public Health, working on behalf of health and local authorities, produce an equity profile for the population they serve, and undertake a triennial audit of progress towards achieving objectives to reduce inequalities in health.

39.1 We recommend there should be a duty of partnership between the NHS Executive and regional government to ensure that effective local partnerships are established between health, local authorities and other agencies and that joint programmes to address health inequalities are in place and monitored.

Effective working will be strengthened by better co-ordination of policies and programmes between Government Departments, non-Departmental public bodies and agencies, such as the Health Education Authority, Food Standards Agency and Environment Agency. This returns us to our first recommendation which emphasises the need for Departments to consider impact assessments on health inequalities in the formulation of policy, and to keep these developments under review.

We RECOMMEND that as part of health impact assessment, all policies likely to have a direct or indirect impact on health should be evaluated in terms of their impact on health inequalities, and should be formulated in such a way that by favouring the less well off they will, wherever possible, reduce such inequalities (recommendation 1).

List of Recommendations

General Recommendations (see pages 29–31)

1. We RECOMMEND that as part of health impact assessment, all policies likely to have a direct or indirect effect on health should be evaluated in terms of their impact on health inequalities, and should be formulated in such a way that by favouring the less well off they will, wherever possible, reduce such inequalities.

1.1 We recommend establishing mechanisms to monitor inequalities in health and to evaluate the effectiveness of measures taken to reduce them.

1.2 We recommend a review of data needs to improve the capacity to monitor inequalities in health and their determinants at a national and local level.

2. We RECOMMEND a high priority is given to policies aimed at improving health and reducing health inequalities in women of childbearing age, expectant mothers and young children.

Poverty, Income, Tax and Benefits (see pages 32–36)

3. We RECOMMEND policies which will further reduce income inequalities, and improve the living standards of households in receipt of social security benefits. Specifically:

3.1 we recommend further reductions in poverty in women of child-bearing age, expectant mothers, young children and older people should be made by increasing benefits in cash or in kind to them.

3.2 We recommend uprating of benefits and pensions according to principles which protect and, where possible, improve the standard of living of those who depend on them and which narrow the gap between their standard of living and average living standards.

3.3 We recommend measures to increase the uptake of benefits in entitled groups.

We recommend further steps to increase employment opportunities (recommendation 8.1)

Education (see pages 36–44)

4. *We RECOMMEND the provision of additional resources for schools serving children from less well off groups to enhance their educational achievement. The Revenue Support Grant formula and other funding mechanisms should be more strongly weighted to reflect need and socioeconomic disadvantage.*

5. *We RECOMMEND the further development of high quality pre-school education so that it meets, in particular, the needs of disadvantaged families. We also recommend that the benefits of pre-school education to disadvantaged families are evaluated and, if necessary, additional resources are made available to support further development.*

6. *We RECOMMEND the further development of "health promoting schools", initially focused on, but not limited to, disadvantaged communities.*

7. *We RECOMMEND further measures to improve the nutrition provided at school, including: the promotion of school food policies; the development of budgeting and cooking skills; the preservation of free school meals entitlement; the provision of free school fruit; and the restriction of less healthy food.*

Employment (see pages 44–50)

8. *We RECOMMEND policies which improve the opportunities for work and which ameliorate the health consequences of unemployment. Specifically:*

8.1 *we recommend further steps to increase employment opportunities.*

8.2 *We recommend further investment in high quality training for young and long-term unemployed people.*

We recommend policies which will further reduce income inequalities, and improve the living standards of households in receipt of social security benefits (recommendation 3).

We recommend an integrated policy for the provision of affordable, high quality day care and pre-school education with extra resources for disadvantaged communities (recommendation 21.1).

9. *We RECOMMEND policies to improve the quality of jobs, and reduce psychosocial work hazards. Specifically:*

9.1 *we recommend employers, unions and relevant agencies take further measures to improve health through good management practices which lead to an increased level of control, variety and appropriate use of skills in the workforce.*

9.2 *We recommend assessing the impact of employment policies on health and inequalities in health* (see also recommendation 1).

Housing and Environment (see pages 50–55)

10. We RECOMMEND policies which improve the availability of social housing for the less well off within a framework of environmental improvement, planning and design which takes into account social networks, and access to goods and services.

11. We RECOMMEND policies which improve housing provision and access to health care for both officially and unofficially homeless people.

12. We RECOMMEND policies which aim to improve the quality of housing. Specifically:

12.1 we recommend policies to improve insulation and heating systems in new and existing buildings in order to reduce further the prevalence of fuel poverty.

12.2 We recommend amending housing and licensing conditions and housing regulations on space and amenity to reduce accidents in the home, including measures to promote the installation of smoke detectors in existing homes.

13. We RECOMMEND the development of policies to reduce the fear of crime and violence, and to create a safe environment for people to live in.

We recommend policies which will further reduce income inequalities, and improve the living standards of households in receipt of social security benefits (recommendation 3).

Mobility, Transport and Pollution (see pages 55–61)

14. We RECOMMEND the further development of a high quality public transport system which is integrated with other forms of transport and is affordable to the user.

15. We RECOMMEND further measures to encourage walking and cycling as forms of transport and to ensure the safe separation of pedestrians and cyclists from motor vehicles.

16. We RECOMMEND further steps to reduce the usage of motor cars to cut the mortality and morbidity associated with motor vehicle emissions.

17. We RECOMMEND further measures to reduce traffic speed, by environmental design and modification of roads, lower speed limits in built up areas, and stricter enforcement of speed limits.

18. We RECOMMEND concessionary fares should be available to pensioners and disadvantaged groups throughout the country, and that local schemes should emulate high quality schemes, such as those of London and the West Midlands.

Nutrition and the Common Agricultural Policy
(see pages 62–67)

19. We RECOMMEND a comprehensive review of the Common Agricultural Policy (CAP)'s impact on health and inequalities in health.

19.1 We recommend strengthening the CAP Surplus Food Scheme to improve the nutritional position of the less well off.

20. We RECOMMEND policies which will increase the availability and accessibility of foodstuffs to supply an adequate and affordable diet. Specifically:

20.1 We recommend the further development of policies which will ensure adequate retail provision of food to those who are disadvantaged.

We recommend policies which will further reduce income inequalities, and improve the living standards of households in receipt of social security benefits (recommendation 3).

We recommend the further development of a high quality public transport system which is integrated with other forms of transport and is affordable to the user (recommendation 14).

20.2 We recommend policies which reduce the sodium content of processed foods, particularly bread and cereals, and which do not incur additional cost to the consumer.

Mothers, Children and Families (see pages 67–77)

21. We RECOMMEND policies which reduce poverty in families with children by promoting the material support of parents; by removing barriers to work for parents who wish to combine work with parenting; and by enabling those who wish to devote full-time to parenting to do so. Specifically:

21.1 we recommend an integrated policy for the provision of affordable, high quality day care and pre-school education with extra resources for disadvantaged communities (see also: recommendation 5).

We recommend further reductions in poverty in women of child-bearing age, expectant mothers, young children and older people should be made by increasing benefits in cash or in kind to them (recommendation 3.1).

We recommend measures to increase the uptake of benefits in entitled groups (recommendation 3.3).

22. We RECOMMEND policies which improve the health and nutrition of women of child-bearing age and their children with priority given to the elimination of food poverty and the prevention and reduction of obesity. Specifically:

We recommend further reductions in poverty in women of child-bearing age, expectant mothers, young children and older people should be made by increasing benefits in cash or in kind to them (recommendation 3.1).

We recommend further measures to improve the nutrition provided at school, including:
the promotion of school food policies; the development of budgeting and cooking skills;
the preservation of free school meals entitlement; the provision of free school fruit; and the
restriction of less healthy food (recommendation 7).

We recommend a comprehensive review of the Common Agricultural Policy (CAP)'s impact on
health and inequalities in health (recommendation 19).

We recommend policies which will increase the availability and accessibility of foodstuffs to
supply an adequate and affordable diet (recommendation 20).

22.1 We recommend policies which increase the prevalence of breastfeeding.

22.2 We recommend the fluoridation of the water supply.

**22.3 We recommend the further development of programmes to help women to give up
smoking before or during pregnancy, and which are focused on the less well off.**

**23. We RECOMMEND policies that promote the social and emotional support for parents
and children. Specifically:**

**23.1 we recommend the further development of the role and capacity of health visitors to
provide social and emotional support to expectant parents, and parents with young
children.**

**23.2 We recommend local authorities identify and address the physical and psychological
health needs of looked-after children.**

Young People and Adults of Working Age (see pages 77–87)

We recommend policies which improve the opportunities for work and which ameliorate the
health consequences of unemployment (recommendation 8).

We recommend policies to improve the quality of jobs, and reduce psychosocial work hazards
(recommendation 9)

**24. We RECOMMEND measures to prevent suicide among young people, especially among
young men and seriously mentally ill people.**

**25. We RECOMMEND policies which promote sexual health in young people and reduce
unwanted teenage pregnancy, including access to appropriate contraceptive services.**

**26. We RECOMMEND policies which promote the adoption of healthier lifestyles,
particularly in respect of factors which show a strong social gradient in prevalence or
consequences. Specifically:**

**26.1 we recommend policies which promote moderate intensity exercise including: further
provision of cycling and walking routes to school, and other environmental modifications
aimed at the safe separation of pedestrians and cyclists from motor vehicles; and safer
opportunities for leisure.**

26.2 *We recommend policies to reduce tobacco smoking including: restricting smoking in public places; abolishing tobacco advertising and promotion; and community, mass media and educational initiatives.*

26.3 *We recommend increases in the real price of tobacco to discourage young people from becoming habitual smokers and to encourage adult smokers to quit. These increases should be introduced in tandem with policies to improve the living standards of low income households and polices to help smokers in these households become and remain ex-smokers.*

26.4 *We recommend making nicotine replacement therapy available on prescription.*

26.5 *We recommend policies which reduce alcohol-related ill health, accidents and violence, including measures which at least maintain the real cost of alcohol.*

Older People (see pages 87–92)

27. **We RECOMMEND policies which will promote the material well being of older people. Specifically:**

we recommend policies which will further reduce income inequalities, and improve the living standards of households in receipt of social security benefits (recommendation 3).

We recommend uprating of benefits and pensions according to principles which protect and, where possible, improve the standard of living of those who depend on them and which narrow the gap between their standard of living and average living standards (recommendation 3.2).

We recommend measures to increase the uptake of benefits among entitled groups. (recommendation 3.3).

28. **We RECOMMEND the quality of homes in which older people live be improved. Specifically:**

we recommend policies to improve insulation and heating systems in new and existing buildings in order to reduce further the prevalence of fuel poverty (recommendation 12.1).

We recommend amending housing and licensing conditions and housing regulations on space and amenity to reduce accidents in the home, including measures to promote the installation of smoke detectors in existing homes (recommendation 12.2).

29. **We RECOMMEND policies which will promote the maintenance of mobility, independence, and social contacts. Specifically:**

we recommend the development of policies to reduce the fear of crime and violence, and to create a safe environment for people to live in (recommendation 13).

We recommend the further development of a high quality public transport system which is integrated with other forms of transport and is affordable to the user (recommendation 14).

We recommend concessionary fares should be available to pensioners and disadvantaged groups throughout the country, and that local schemes should emulate high quality schemes, such as those of London and the West Midlands (recommendation 18).

30. We RECOMMEND the further development of health and social services for older people, so that these services are accessible and distributed according to need.

We recommend a review of data needs to improve the capacity to monitor inequalities in health and their determinants at a national and local level (recommendation 1.2).

Ethnicity (see pages 92–100)

31. We RECOMMEND that the needs of minority ethnic groups are specifically considered in the development and implementation of policies aimed at reducing socioeconomic inequalities. Specifically:

we recommend policies which will further reduce income inequalities, and improve the living standards of households in receipt of social security benefits (recommendation 3).

We recommend policies which improve the opportunities for work and which ameliorate the health consequences of unemployment (recommendation 8)

We recommend policies which improve the availability of social housing for the less well off within a framework of environmental improvement, planning and design which takes into account social networks, and access to goods and services (recommendation 10).

We recommend policies which aim to improve the quality of housing (recommendation 12).

We recommend the development of policies to reduce the fear of crime and violence, and to create a safe environment for people to live in (recommendation 13).

We recommend the further development of a high quality public transport system which is integrated with other forms of transport and is affordable to the user (recommendation 14).

We recommend further measures to encourage walking and cycling as forms of transport and to ensure the safe separation of pedestrians and cyclists from motor vehicles (recommendation 15).

We recommend further steps to reduce the usage of motor cars to cut the mortality and morbidity associated with motor vehicle emissions (recommendation 16).

We recommend further measures to reduce traffic speed, by environmental design and modification of roads, lower speed limits in built up areas, and stricter enforcement of speed limits (recommendation 17).

We recommend concessionary fares should be available to pensioners and disadvantaged groups throughout the country, and that local schemes should emulate high quality schemes, such as those of London and the West Midlands (recommendation 18)

32. We RECOMMEND the further development of services which are sensitive to the needs of minority ethnic people and which promote greater awareness of their health risks.

33. **We RECOMMEND the needs of minority ethnic groups are specifically considered in needs assessment, resource allocation, health care planning and provision. Specifically:**

we recommend a review of data needs to improve the capacity to monitor inequalities in health and their determinants at a national and local level (recommendation 1.2).

Gender (see pages 100–110)

34. **We RECOMMEND policies which reduce the excess mortality from accidents and suicide in young men (see also: recommendation 24). Specifically:**

we recommend policies which improve the opportunities for work and which ameliorate the health consequences of unemployment (recommendation 8).

We recommend policies which improve housing provision and access to health care for both officially and unofficially homeless people (recommendation 11).

We recommend further measures to encourage walking and cycling as forms of transport and to ensure the safe separation of pedestrians and cyclists from motor vehicles (recommendation 15).

We recommend further steps to reduce the usage of motor cars to cut the mortality and morbidity associated with motor vehicle emissions (recommendation 16).

We recommend further measures to reduce traffic speed, by environmental design and modification of roads, lower speed limits in built up areas, and stricter enforcement of speed limits (recommendation 17).

We recommend measures to prevent suicide among young people, especially among young men and seriously mentally ill people (recommendation 24).

We recommend policies which reduce alcohol-related ill health, accidents and violence, including measures which at least maintain the real cost of alcohol (recommendation 26.5).

35. **We RECOMMEND policies which reduce psychosocial ill health in young women in disadvantaged circumstances, particularly those caring for young children. Specifically:**

we recommend further reductions in poverty in women of child-bearing age, expectant mothers, young children and older people should be made by increasing benefits in cash or in kind to them (recommendation 3.1).

We recommend uprating of benefits and pensions according to principles which protect and, where possible, improve the standard of living of those who depend on them, and which narrow the gap between their standard of living and average living standards (recommendation 3.2).

We recommend measures to increase the uptake of benefits among entitled groups (recommendation 3.3).

We recommend policies which improve the availability of social housing for the less well off within a framework of environmental improvement, planning and design which takes into account social networks, and access to goods and services (recommendation 10).

We recommend the further development of a high quality public transport system which is integrated with other forms of transport and is affordable to the user (recommendation 14).

We recommend policies which will increase the availability and accessibility of foodstuffs to supply an adequate and affordable diet (recommendation 20).

We recommend policies which reduce poverty in families with children by promoting the material support of parents; by removing barriers to work for parents who wish to combine work with parenting, and by enabling those who wish to devote full-time to parenting to do so (recommendation 21).

We recommend an integrated policy for the provision of affordable, high quality day care and pre-school education with extra resources for disadvantaged communities. (recommendation 21.1).

We recommend policies which improve the health and nutrition of women of child-bearing age and their children with priority given to the elimination of food poverty and the prevention and reduction of obesity (recommendation 22).

We recommend policies which promote the social and emotional support for parents and children (recommendation 23).

We recommend the further development of the role and capacity of health visitors to provide social and emotional support to expectant parents, and parents with young children (recommendation 23.1).

We recommend policies which promote sexual health in young people and reduce unwanted teenage pregnancy, including access to appropriate contraceptive services (recommendation 25).

36. We RECOMMEND policies which reduce disability and ameliorate its consequences in older women, particularly those living alone. Specifically:

we recommend further reductions in poverty in women of child-bearing age, expectant mothers, young children and older people should be made by increasing benefits in cash or in kind to them (recommendation 3.1).

We recommend uprating of benefits and pensions according to principles which protect and, where possible, improve the standard of living of those who depend on them, and which narrow the gap between their standard of living and average living standards (recommendation 3.2).

We recommend measures to increase the uptake of benefits among entitled groups (recommendation 3.3).

We recommend the development of policies to reduce the fear of crime and violence, and to create a safe environment for people to live in (recommendation 13).

We recommend the further development of a high quality public transport system which is integrated with other forms of transport and is affordable to the user (recommendation 14)

We recommend concessionary fares should be available to pensioners and disadvantaged groups throughout the country, and that local schemes should emulate high quality schemes, such as those of London and the West Midlands (recommendation 18).

We recommend the quality of homes in which older people live be improved (recommendation 28).

We recommend the further development of health and social sevices for older people, so that these services are accessible and distributed according to need (recommendation 30).

The National Health Service (pages 111–119)

37. We RECOMMEND that providing equitable access to effective care in relation to need should be a governing principle of all policies in the NHS. Priority should be given to the achievement of equity in the planning, implementation and delivery of services at every level of the NHS. Specifically:

37.1 we recommend extending the focus of clinical governance to give equal prominence to equity of access to effective health care.

37.2 We recommend extending the remit of the National Institute for Clinical Excellence to include equity of access to effective health care.

37.3 We recommend developing the National Service Frameworks to address inequities in access to effective primary care.

37.4 We recommend that performance management in relation to the national performance management framework is focused on achieving more equitable access, provision and targeting of effective services in relation to need in both primary and hospital sectors.

37.5 We recommend that the Department of Health and NHS Executive set out their responsibilities for furthering the principle of equity of access to effective health and social care, and that health authorities, working with Primary Care Groups and providers on local clinical governance, agree priorities and objectives for reducing inequities in access to effective care. These should form part of the Health Improvement Programme.

38. We RECOMMEND giving priority to the achievement of a more equitable allocation of NHS resources. This will require adjustments to the ways in which resources are allocated and the speed with which resource allocation targets are met. Specifically:

38.1 we recommend reviewing the "pace of change" policy to enable health authorities that are furthest from their capitation targets to move more quickly to their actual target.

38.2 We recommend extending the principle of needs-based weighting to non-cash limited General Medical Services (GMS) resources. The size and effectiveness of deprivation payments in meeting the needs and improving the health outcomes amongst the most disadvantaged populations, including ethnic minorities should be assessed.

38.3 We recommend reviewing the size and effectiveness of the Hospital and Community Health Service (HCHS) formula and deprivation payments in influencing the health care outcomes of the most disadvantaged populations, and to consider alternative methods of focusing resources for health promotion and public health care to reduce health inequalities.

38.4 We recommend establishing a review of the relationship of private practice to the NHS with particular reference to access to effective treatments, resource allocation and availability of staff.

39. We RECOMMEND Directors of Public Health, working on behalf of health and local authorities, produce an equity profile for the population they serve, and undertake a triennial audit of progress towards achieving objectives to reduce inequalities in health.

39.1 We recommend there should be a duty of partnership between the NHS Executive and regional government to ensure that effective local partnerships are established between health, local authorities and other agencies and that joint programmes to address health inequalities are in place and monitored.

We RECOMMEND that as part of health impact assessment, all policies likely to have a direct or indirect effect on health should be evaluated in terms of their impact on health inequalities, and should be formulated in such a way that by favouring the less well off they will, wherever possible, reduce such inequalities (recommendation 1).

References

1   Department of Health. *Our healthier nation: a contract for health.* London: The Stationery Office, 1998.

2   Scottish Office Department of Health. *Working together for a healthier Scotland: a consultation document.* Edinburgh: The Stationery Office, 1998.

3   Secretary of State for Wales. *Better health, better Wales: a consultative paper.* Cardiff: Welsh Office, 1998.

4   Department of Health and Social Services. *Well into 2000: a positive agenda for health and wellbeing.* Belfast: The Stationery Office, 1997.

5   Department of Health. *The new NHS – modern and dependable.* London: The Stationery Office, 1997.

6   Whitehead M. Life and death over the millennium. In: Drever F, Whitehead M, eds. *Health inequalities: decennial supplement: DS Series no.15.* London: The Stationery Office, 1997.

7   Farr W. *Letter to the Registrar General on the years 1851–1860: supplement to the 25th report of the Registrar General.* London: General Register Office, 1864.

8   Beveridge W. *Social insurance and allied services.* London: HMSO, 1942.

9   Black D, Morris J, Smith C, Townsend P. *Inequalities in health: report of a Research Working Group.* London: Department of Health and Social Security, 1980.

10 Townsend P, Whitehead M, Davidson N. Introduction to inequalities in health. In: Townsend P, Whitehead M, Davidson N, eds. *Inequalities in health: the Black Report and the Health Divide.* 2nd edition. London: Penguin, 1992.

11 World Health Organisation. *Targets for health for all.* Copenhagen: World Health Organisation, 1985.

12 Whitehead M. The Health Divide. In: Townsend P, Whitehead M, Davidson N, eds. *Inequalities in health: the Black Report and the Health Divide.* 2nd edition. London: Penguin, 1992.

13 Department of Health. *Variations in health: what can the Department of Health and NHS do?* London: Department of Health, 1995.

14 Benzeval M, Judge K, Whitehead M, eds. *Tackling inequalities in health: an agenda for action.* London: Kings Fund, 1995.

15 Dahlgren G, Whitehead M. *Policies and strategies to promote social equity in health.* Stockholm: Institute of Futures Studies, 1991.

16 Whitehead M. Tackling inequalities: a review of policy initiatives. In: Benzeval M, Judge K, Whitehead M, eds. *Tackling inequalities in health: an agenda for action.* London: Kings Fund, 1995.

17 House of Commons. Parliamentary debate. Oral Answers. *Hansard* 1997;**295**:Column 1139–1140.

18 Hsieh C, Pugh M. Poverty, income inequality and violent crime: a meta-analysis of recent aggregate data studies. *Criminal Justice Review* 1993;**18**:182–202.

19 Wilkinson R, Kawachi I, Kennedy B. Mortality, the social environment, crime and violence. In: Bartley M, Blane D, Davey Smith G, eds. *Sociology of health inequalities.* Oxford: Blackwell, 1998.

20 Kuh D, Ben-Shlomo Y, eds. *A life course approach to chronic disease epidemiology.* Oxford: Oxford University Press, 1997.

21 Barker D. *Mothers, babies and health in later life.* Edinburgh: Churchill Livingstone, 1998.

22 Whitehead M, Diderichsen F. International evidence on social inequalities in health. In: Drever F, Whitehead M, eds. *Health inequalities: decennial supplement: DS Series no.15.* London: The Stationery Office, 1997.

23 Illsley R, Baker D. *Inequalities in health: adapting the theory to fit the facts.* Bath: University of Bath, Centre for the Analysis of Social Policy, 1997.

24 General Register Office. *59th Annual Report of the Registrar General. Births, deaths and marriages in England –1896.* London: HMSO, 1898.

25 Office for National Statistics. *Mortality statistics: cause 1996, series DH2, no.23.* London: The Stationery Office, 1998.

26 Office for National Statistics. *English life tables, no 15.* London: The Stationery Office, 1997.

27 Bebbington A, Carton R. *Healthy life expectancy in England and Wales: recent evidence.* Canterbury: Personal Social Services Research Unit, 1996.

28 Office for National Statistics. *Living in Britain: results from the general household survey '96.* London: The Stationery Office, 1998.

29 Drever F, Bunting J. Patterns and trends in male mortality. In: Drever F, Whitehead M, eds. *Health inequalities: decennial supplement: DS Series no.15.* London: The Stationery Office, 1997.

30 Harding S, Bethune A, Maxwell R, Brown J. Mortality trends using the longitudinal study. In: Drever F, Whitehead M, eds. *Health inequalities: decennial supplement: DS Series no.15.* London: The Stationery Office, 1997.

31 Hattersly L. Expectation of life by social class. In: Drever F, Whitehead M, eds. *Health inequalities: decennial supplement.* London: The Stationery Office, 1997.

32 Office for National Statistics. *Unpublished analysis.* 1998.

33 Blane D, Drever F. Inequality among men in standardised years of potential life, 1970–93. *British Medical Journal* 1998;**317**:255–260.

34 Office for National Statistics. *Series DH3 mortality statistics: perinatal and infant: social and biological factors.* London: The Stationery Office, 1997.

35 Colhoun H, Prescott-Clarke P. *Health Survey for England 1994.* London: HMSO, 1996.

36 Prescott-Clarke P, Primatesta P. *Health Survey for England 1995.* London: The Stationery Office, 1997.

37 Prescott-Clarke P, Primatesta P. *Health Survey for England '96.* London: The Stationery Office, 1998.

38 Meltzer H, Gill B, Petticrew M, Hinds K. *The prevalence of psychiatric morbidity among adults living in private households.* London: Office of Population Censuses and Surveys/HMSO, 1995.

39 Church J, Whyman S. A review of recent social and economic trends. In: Drever F, Whitehead M, eds. *Health inequalities: decennial supplement: DS Series no.15.* London: The Stationery Office, 1997.

40 Office for National Statistics. *Social Trends 28, 1998 edition.* London: The Stationery Office, 1998.

41 Office for National Statistics. *Regional trends, no.32.* London: The Stationery Office, 1997.

42 Office for National Statistics. *Social Trends 27, 1997 edition.* London: The Stationery Office, 1997.

43 Office for National Statistics. *Labour market statistics release.* London: Office for National Statistics, 1998.

44 Philpott J. Unemployment, inequality and inefficiency. The incidence and costs of unemployment. In: Glynn T, Miliband D, eds. *Paying for inequality: the economic costs of social injustice.* London: Rivers Oram Press, 1994.

45 Office for National Statistics. *Economic Trends no. 533.* London: The Stationery Office, 1998.

46 Department of the Environment. *Housing policy: technical volume part 1.* London: HMSO, 1977.

47 Department of the Environment, Transport and the Regions. *Housing and construction statistics, Great Britain, March quarter 1998: part 2 no 73*. London: The Stationery Office, 1998.

48 Office for National Statistics. *Housing in England 1995/96. A report of the 1995/96 survey of English housing carried out by the Social Survey Divison of Office for National Statistics on behalf of the Department of Environment*. London: The Stationery Office, 1997.

49 Department of the Environment. *Projection of households in England to 2016*. London: HMSO, 1995.

50 Department of the Environment, Transport and the Regions. *English house condition survey 1996*. London: The Stationery Office, 1998.

51 Department of the Environment, Transport and the Regions. *Local authority activities under the homeless legislation, England: fourth quarter 1997*. London: Department of the Environment, Transport and the Regions, 1998.

52 Office of Population Censuses and Surveys. *1991 Census: housing and availability of cars*. London: HMSO, 1993.

53 Office for National Statistics. *Living in Britain: results from the general household survey 1995*. London: The Stationery Office, 1997.

54 Office for National Statistics. *1991 Census: key statistics for urban and rural areas, Great Britain*. London: The Stationery Office, 1997.

55 Ministry of Agriculture, Fisheries and Food. *National food survey 1980–1996*. London: HMSO, various years.

56 Department of Health. *The diets of British schoolchildren*. London: HMSO, 1989.

57 Gregory J, Foster K, Tyler H, Wiseman M. *The dietary and nutritional survey of British adults*. London: HMSO, 1990.

58 Gregory J, Collins D, Davies P, Hughes J, Clarke P. *National Diet and Nutrition Survey: Children aged 1½ to 4½ years*. London: HMSO, 1995.

59 Foster K, Lader D, Cheesbrough S. *Infant feeding 1995*. London: The Stationery Office, 1997.

60 Charlton J, Wallace M, White M. Long-term illness: results from the 1991 Census. *Population Trends* 1994;**75**:18–25.

61 Wild S, McKeigue P. Cross-sectional analysis of mortality by country of birth in England and Wales, 1970–92. *British Medical Journal* 1997; **314**:705–710.

62 Botting B. Mortality in childhood. In: Drever F, Whitehead M, eds. *Health inequalities: decennial supplement: DS Series,no.15*. London: The Stationery Office, 1997.

63 Office for National Statistics. *Smoking in secondary school children*. London: HMSO/The Stationery Office, various years.

64 Evaluation Group. Report to the Independent Inquiry into Inequalities in Health. 1998.

65 Hills J. *Income and wealth: the latest evidence*. York: Joseph Rowntree Foundation, 1998.

66 Modood T, Berthoud R, Lakey J, et al. *Ethnic minorities in Britain: diversity and disadvantage*. London: Policy Studies Institute, 1997.

67 Department of Social Security. *Family resources survey, Great Britain, 1993/4*. London: HMSO, 1995.

68 Berthoud R. *Disability benefits: a review of the issues and options for reform*. York: Joseph Rowntree Foundation, 1998.

69 Berthoud R, Lakey J, McKay S. *The economic problems of disabled people*. London: Policy Studies Institute, 1993.

70 Walker R, Park J. Unpicking poverty. In: Oppenheim C, ed. *An inclusive society: strategies for tackling poverty*. London: Institute for Public Policy Research, 1998.

71 Department of Social Security. *Social Security 1996 statistics*. London: The Stationery Office, 1996.

72 Department of Social Security. *Households below average income: a statistical analysis 1979–1994/95*. London: The Stationery Office, 1997.

73 Drever F, Megens T. *Unpublished analysis*. 1998.

74 Office for National Statistics. *General household survey: unpublished analysis*. 1997.

75 Giles C, Johnson P. Tax reform in the UK and changes in the progressivity of the tax system 1985–1995. *Fiscal Studies* 1994;**15**:64–86.

76 Oppenheim C, Harker L. *Poverty: the facts.* London: Child Poverty Action Group, 1996.

77 Department of Social Security. *Social Security 1997 statistics.* London: The Stationery Office, 1997.

78 Berthoud R, Ford R. *Relative needs overview of an analysis of variations in the living standards of different types of household.* London: Policy Studies Institute, 1996.

79 Eardley T. *Social assistance in OECD countries: a study carried out on behalf of the Department of Social Security and the OECD by the Social Policy Research Unit.* London: HMSO, 1996.

80 Bradshaw J. *Budget standards for the UK.* Aldershot: Avebury, 1993.

81 Oldfield N, Yu A. *The cost of a child: living standards for the 1990s.* London: Child Poverty Action Group, 1993.

82 Middleton S, Ashworth K, Walker R. *Family fortunes.* London: Child Poverty Action Group, 1994.

83 Dallison J, Lobstein T. *Poor expectations: poverty and undernourishment in pregnancy.* London: NCH Action for Children and The Maternity Alliance, 1995.

84 Middleton S, Ashworth K, Braithwaite I. *Small fortunes: spending on children, childhood poverty and parental sacrifice.* York: Joseph Rowntree Foundation, 1997.

85 Bradshaw J. *Household budgets and living standards.* York: Joseph Rowntree Foundation, 1993.

86 Department of Social Security. *Income related benefits: estimates of take-up in 1995/96.* London: Department of Social Security, 1998.

87 Department of Social Security. *New ambitions for our country – a new contract for welfare.* London: The Stationery Office, 1998.

88 Walker R. Positive welfare. *New Economics* 1998;**5**:69–128.

89 Van Oorschot W. *Realising rights.* London: Avebury, 1995.

90 NHS Centre for Reviews and Dissemination. *Review of the research on the effectiveness of health service interventions to reduce variations in health.* York: University of York, 1995.

91 Kehrer B, Wolin V. Impact of income maintenance on low birthweight, evidence from the Gary experiment. *Journal of Human Resources* 1979;**14**:434–462.

92 Kempson E, Bryson A, Rowlingson K. *Hard times? How poor families make ends meet.* London: Policy Studies Institute, 1994.

93 Dobson B, Beardsworth A, Keil T, Walker R. *Diet, choice and poverty: social, cultural and nutritional aspects of food consumption among low income families.* Loughborough: Loughborough University of Technology, Centre for Research in Social Policy, 1994.

94 Dowler E, Calvert C. *Nutrition and diet in lone-parent families in London.* London: Family Policy Studies Centre, 1995.

95 Lobstein T. *The nutrition of women on low income.* London: Food Commission, 1991.

96 Markus T. Cold, condensation and housing poverty. In: Burridge R, Ormandy D, eds. *Unhealthy housing: research, remedies and reform.* London: E. and F.N. Spon, 1993.

97 Savage A. *Warmth in winter: evaluation of an information pack for elderly people.* Cardiff: University of Wales College of Medicine Research Team for the Care of the Elderly, 1988.

98 Drever F, Whitehead M, eds. *Health inequalities: decennial supplement: DS Series no.15.* London: The Stationery Office, 1997.

99 Tones K. The health promoting school: some reflections on evaluation. *Health Education Research* 1996;**11**:R1–R8.

100 Dahlgren G, Whitehead M. *Policies and strategies to promote equity in health.* Copenhagen: World Health Organisation, 1992.

101 World Health Organisation. *The European network of health promoting schools: a joint World Health Organisation (Europe) and Commission of the European Communities and Council of Europe project.* Copenhagen: Commission of the European Communities and Council of Europe, 1993.

102 Social Exclusion Unit. *Truancy and school exclusion: report by the Social Exclusion Unit.* London: The Stationery Office, 1998.

103 Thomas G. *Exam performance in special schools.* Bristol: Centre for Studies on Inclusive Education, 1997.

104 Montgomery S, Schoon I. Health and health behaviour. In: Bynner J, Ferri E, Shepherd P, eds. *Twentysomething in the 1990s: getting on, getting by, getting nowhere.* Aldershot: Ashgate, 1997.

105 Bynner J, Parsons S. *It doesn't get any better: the impact of poor basic skills on the lives of 37 year olds.* London: The Basic Skills Agency, 1997.

106 Marmot M, Ryff C, Bumpass L, Shipley M, Marks N. Social inequalities in health: next questions and converging evidence. *Social Science and Medicine* 1997;**44**:901–910.

107 Wadsworth M. Family and education as determinants of health. In: Blane D, Brunner E, Wilkinson R, eds. *Health and social organisation: towards a health policy for the 21st century.* London: Routledge, 1996.

108 Wadsworth M. Changing social factors and their long-term implications for health. *British Medical Bulletin* 1997;**53**:198–209.

109 Glennerster H. Education: reaping the harvest? In: Glennerster H, Hills J, eds. *The state of welfare: the economics of social spending.* Oxford: Oxford University Press, 1998.

110 Thomas S, Mortimore P. Comparison of value-added models for secondary-school effectiveness. *Research Papers in Education* 1996;**11**:5–33.

111 Ball C, ed. *Start right: the importance of early learning.* London: Royal Society of Arts, 1994.

112 Meltzer H. *Day care services for children: a survey carried out on behalf of the Department of Health in 1990.* London: HMSO, 1994.

113 Zoritch B, Roberts I. The health and welfare effects of day care for pre-school children: a systematic review of randomised controlled trials. In: The Cochrane Database of Systematic Reviews, ed. *The Cochrane Library, Issue 2, 1998.* Oxford: Update Software (updated quarterly), 1998.

114 Sylva K. The early years curriculum: evidence based proposals. In: School Curriculum and Assessment Authority, ed. *Developing the primary school curriculum: the next steps.* London: School Curriculum and Assessment Authority, 1997.

115 Sylva K. The impact of early learning on children's later development. In: Ball C, ed. *Start right: the importance of early learning.* London: Royal Society of Arts, 1994.

116 Leather S. *The making of modern malnutrition: an overview of food poverty in the UK.* London: Caroline Walker Trust, 1996.

117 Health Education Authority. *Tomorrow's young adults.* London: Health Education Authority, 1990.

118 Glendinning A, Schucksmith J, Hendry L. Social class and adolescent smoking behaviour. *Social Science and Medicine* 1994;**38**:1449–60.

119 Green G, Macintyre S, West P, Ecob R. Like parent like child? Associations between drinking and smoking behaviour of parents and their children. *British Journal of Addiction* 1991;**86**:745–58.

120 Hamilton K, Saunders L. *The health promoting school: a summary of the European Network of Health Promoting Schools evaluation project in England.* London: Health Education Authority/National Foundation for Educational Research, 1997.

121 Division of Mental Health. *Life skills education in schools.* Geneva: World Health Organisation, 1993.

122 Bierman KL. Process of change during social skills training with pre-adolescents and its relation to treatment outcomes. *Child Development* 1986;**57**:230–240.

123 Pelligrini D. Training in interpersonal cognitive problem-solving. In: Rutter M, Taylor E, Hersov L, eds. *Child and adolescent psychiatry: modern approaches.* Oxford: Blackwell, 1994.

124 Hope P, Sharland P. *Tomorrow's parents: developing parenthood education in schools.* London: Calouste Gulbenkian Foundation, 1997.

125 Hawkins J, Catalan R, Morrison D, O'Donnell J, Abbot R, Day L. The Seattle Social Development Project: Effects of the first four years on proactive factors and problem behaviours. In: McCord J, Tremblay R, eds. *Preventing antisocial behaviour.* New York: Guildford Press, 1992.

126 Kellam S, Rebok G. Building developmental and etiological theory through epidemiological based preventive intervention trials. In: McCord J, Tremblay RE, eds. *Preventing antisocial behaviour*. New York: Guildford Press, 1992.

127 White D, Pitts M. *Health promotion with young people for the prevention of substance misuse*. London: Health Education Authority, 1997.

128 Hurry J, Lloyd C. *A follow up evaluation of Project Charlie: a life skills drug education programme for primary schools*. Paper 16. London: Home Office Drug Prevention Unit, 1997.

129 UNAIDS. *Impact of HIV and sexual health education on the sexual behaviour of young people: a review update*. Geneva: UNAIDS, 1997.

130 NHS Centre for Reviews and Dissemination. Preventing and reducing the adverse effects of unintended teenage pregnancies. *Effective Health Care* 1997;**3.**

131 Gregory J, Collins D, Davies P, Hughes J, Clark P. *National Diet and Nutrition Survey: Children aged $1^1/_2$ to $4^1/_2$ years: volume 1*. London: HMSO, 1995.

132 Department for Education and Employment. *Statistical returns 1997*. 1998.

133 Department for Education and Employment. *Eating well at school*. London: Department for Education and Employment, 1998.

134 Jahoda M. *Employment and unemployment*. Cambridge: Cambridge University Press, 1982.

135 Smith R. *Unemployment and health: a disaster and a challenge*. Oxford: Oxford University Press, 1987.

136 Sly F. Disability and the labour market. *Labour Market Trends* 1996;**September**:413–24.

137 Lawless P, Martin R, Hardy S. *Unemployment and social exclusion: landscapes of labour inequality*. London: Jessica Kingsley Publishers, 1998.

138 Nickell S, Bell B. The collapse in demand for the unskilled and unemployment across the OECD. *Oxford review of economic policy: unemployment* 1995;**11**:40–62.

139 Payne J, Payne C. Trends in job loss and recruitment in Britain 1979–1991. In: White M, ed. *Unemployment and public policy in a changing labour market*. London: Policy Studies Institute, 1994.

140 Bartley M. Unemployment and health: understanding the relationship. *Journal of Epidemiology and Community Health* 1994;**48**:333–7.

141 Shortt S. Is unemployment pathogenic? A review of current concepts with lessons for policy planners. *International Journal of Health Services* 1996;**26**:569–589.

142 Bethune A. Unemployment and mortality. In: Drever F, Whitehead M, eds. *Health inequalities: decennial supplement: DS Series no.15*. London: The Stationery Office, 1997.

143 Moser K, Goldblatt P, Fox J, Jones D. Unemployment and mortality. In: Goldblatt P, ed. *Longitudinal study 1971–1981: mortality and social organisation*. London: HMSO, 1990.

144 Daniel W. *The unemployment flow*. London: Policy Studies Institute, 1990.

145 Moylan S, Millar J, Davies R. *For richer, for poorer? Department of Health and Social Security cohort study of unemployed men*. London: HMSO, 1984.

146 White H. *Long-term unemployment and labour markets*. London: Policy Studies Institute, 1983.

147 Piachaud D. A price worth paying? The costs of unemployment. In: Philpott J, ed. *Working for full employment*. London: Routledge, 1997.

148 Berthoud R. *The reform of supplementary benefit*. London: Policy Studies Institute, 1984.

149 White H. *Against unemployment*. London: Policy Studies Institute, 1991.

150 Bradshaw J. *Child poverty and deprivation in the UK*. London: National Children's Bureau, 1990.

151 Kumar V. *Poverty and inequality in the UK*. London: National Children's Bureau, 1993.

152 Montgomery S, Bartley M, Cook D, Wadsworth M. Health and social precursors of unemployment in young men in Great Britain. *Journal of Epidemiology and Community Health* 1996;**50**:415–422.

153 Wadsworth M. *The imprint of time: childhood, history and adult life*. Oxford: Oxford University Press, 1991.

154 Sly F, Duxbury R, Tillsley C. Disability and the labour market: findings from the Labour Force Survey. *Labour Market Trends* 1995;**December**:439–57.

155 The Carnegie United Kingdom Trust. *The Carnegie Young People Initiative: years of decision.* Leicester: Youth Work Press, 1996.

156 Chatrick B, Maclagan I. *Taking their chances: education, training and employment opportunities for young people.* London: The Children's Society, 1995.

157 Dolton P, Makepeace G, Treble J. The Youth Training Scheme and the School-to-Work transition. *Oxford Economic Papers* 1994;**46**:629–657.

158 Lindley R. *The School-to-Work transition in the United Kingdom.* London: International Labour Review, 1996.

159 Maclagan I. *A broken promise: the failure of youth training policy.* London: Youthaid and The Children's Society, 1992.

160 Rolfe H, Bryson A, Metcalf H. *The effectiveness of Training and Enterprise Councils in achieving jobs and qualifications for disadvantaged groups: Department for Education and Employment research study 4.* London: HMSO, 1996.

161 Dennehy A, Smith L, Harker P. *Not to be ignored: young people, poverty and health.* London: Child Poverty Action Group, 1997.

162 Annabel Jackson Associates. *Foyers: the step in the right direction.* London: Foyer Federation, 1996.

163 Chatrick B. *Foyers: a home and a job?* London: Youthaid, 1994.

164 Bradshaw J, Kennedy S, Kilkey M, et al. *The employment of lone parents: a comparison of policy in 20 countries.* London: Family Policy Studies Centre, 1996.

165 Department of Trade and Industry. *Fairness at work.* London: The Stationery Office, 1998.

166 Gregg P, Wadsworth J. A short history of labour turnover, job tenure and job security. *Oxford review of economic policy: unemployment* 1995;**11**:73–90.

167 Martin R. Regional dimensions of Europe's unemployment crisis. In: Lawless P, Martin R, Hardy S, eds. *Unemployment and social exclusion: landscapes of labour inequality.* London: Jessica Kingsley Publishers, 1998.

168 Pollert A. *Fairwell to flexibility.* Oxford: Basil Blackwell, 1998.

169 Prescott-Clarke P. *Employment and handicap.* London: Social and Community Planning Research, 1990.

170 Health and Safety Executive. *Self-reported work-related illness in 1995: results from a household survey.* London: Health and Safety Executive Books, 1998.

171 Hemingway H, Marmot M. Psychosocial factors in the aetiology and prognosis of coronary heart disease: a systematic review of prospective cohort studies. In: Yusuf S, Cairns JA, Camm AJ, Fallen EL, Gersh BJ, eds. *Evidence based cardiology.* London: BMJ Books, 1998.

172 Marmot M, Bosma H, Hemingway H, Brunner E, Stansfield S. Contributions of job control and other risk factors to social variations in coronary heart disease incidence. *Lancet* 1997;**350**:235–239.

173 Hemingway H, Shipley M, Stansfield S, Marmot M. Sickness absence from back pain, psychosocial work characteristics and employment grade among office workers. *Scandinavian Journal of Work, Environment and Health* 1997;**23**:121–9.

174 Emdad R, Belkic K, Theorell T, Cizinsky S, Savic C, Olsson K. Psychophysiologic sensitization to headlight glare among professional drivers with and without cardiovascular disease. *Journal of Occupational Health Psychology* 1998;**3**:147–160.

175 Siegrist J. Adverse health effects of high effort/low reward conditions. *Journal of Occupational Health Psychology* 1996;**1**:27–41.

176 Karasek R, Theorell T. *Healthy work.* New York: Basic Books, 1990.

177 Karasek R. Stress prevention through work reorganization: a summary of 19 international case studies. In: International Labour Organisation, ed. *Preventing stress at work: conditions of work digest, volume II, no 2.* Geneva: International Labour Organisation, 1992.

178 World Health Organisation. *Health promotion in the workplace: strategy options. European Health Series No.10.* Copenhagen: World Health Organisation, 1995.

179 Health and Safety Executive. *Stress at work: a guide for employers*. London: Health and Safety Executive Books, 1995.

180 Health and Safety Executive. *Mental well-being in the workplace: a resource pack for management training and development*. London: Health and Safety Executive Books, 1998.

181 Levi L. Managing stress in work settings at the national level in Sweden. In: International Labour Organisation, ed. *Preventing stress at work: conditions of work digest, volume II, no 2*. Geneva: International Labour Organisation, 1992.

182 Burrows R. *The changing population in social housing in England: contemporary patterns of residential mobility in relation to social housing in England, York*. York: University of York, Centre for Housing Policy, 1997.

183 Wilcox S. *Joseph Rowntree Foundation: housing finance review*. York: Joseph Rowntree Foundation, 1997.

184 Victor C. The health of homeless people: a review. *European Journal of Public Health* 1997;**7**:398–404.

185 Evans A. *"We don't choose to be homeless": Report of the National Inquiry into Preventing Youth Homelessness*. London: Campaign for the Homeless and Rootless, 1996.

186 Shaw M. *A place apart: the spatial polarisation of mortality in Brighton*. Bristol: University of Bristol, 1998.

187 Craig T, Hodson S, Woodward S, Richardson S. *Off to a bad start: a longitudinal study of homeless young people in London*. London: Mental Health Foundation, 1996.

188 Barry A, Carr-Hill R, Glanville J. *Homelessness and health: what do we know? what should be done?* York: University of York, 1991.

189 Stern R, Stilwell B, Heuston J. *From the margins to the mainstream: collaboration in planning services with single homeless people*. London: West Lambeth Health Authority, 1989.

190 Klee H, Reid P. Drug use among young homeless: coping through self-medication. *Health* 1998;**2**:115–134.

191 Bines W. *The health of single homeless people: housing research finding no. 128*. York: Joseph Rowntree Foundation, 1994.

192 British Medical Association. *Deprivation and ill-health – British Medical Association Board of Science and Education Discussion Paper*. London: British Medical Association, 1987.

193 Anderson I, Kemp P, Quilgars D. *Single homeless people*. London: HMSO, 1993.

194 Constantinides P. Safe at home? Children's accidents and inequality. *Radical Community Medicine* 1988;**Spring**:31–3.

195 Child Accident Prevention Trust. *Basic principles of child accident prevention*. London: Child Accident Prevention Trust, 1989.

196 Mental Health Foundation. *Too many for the road: report to the Mental Health Foundation working group on persistent street drinkers*. London: Mental Health Foundation, 1996.

197 Ryan T, Ramprogus S. Current health and social care issues in a community detoxification centre. *Health and Social Care* 1995;**3**:99–104.

198 Flory P, MacGregor S. *Who's vulnerable? The impact of the transition to community care on the drug and alcohol residential sector in England*. London: Alcohol Concern/Standing Conference on Drug Abuse, 1994.

199 Alcohol Concern. *Alcohol in the system? How community care has changed the work of alcohol agencies*. London: Alcohol Concern, 1997.

200 Maclennan D, Meen G, Gibb K, Stephens M. *Fixed commitments, uncertain incomes: sustainable owner-occupation and the economy*. York: Joseph Rowntree Foundation, 1997.

201 Holmans A. Housing demand and need in England to 2011. In: Breheny M, Hall P, eds. *The people: where will they go?* London: The Town and Country Planning Association, 1996.

202 Hills J. *New inequalities*. Cambridge: Cambridge University Press, 1996.

203 Carr J. *Housing research news, volume 2, no.1*. Washington: Office of Housing Research, Fannie Mae, 1993.

204 Kasarda J. *Inner city concentrated poverty in neighbourhood distress, 1970–1990*. Chapel Hill: University of North Carolina, 1993.

205 Newman S. *Last in line: housing assistance for households with children*. Baltimore: Johns Hopkins University, 1993.

206 Gibson T. *Meadowell community development*. Telford: Neighbourhood Initiatives Foundation, 1993.

207 Thake S, Staubach R. *Investing in people: rescuing communities from the margin*. York: Joseph Rowntree Foundation, 1993.

208 Best R. The housing dimension. In: Benzeval M, Judge K, Whitehead M, eds. *Tackling inequalities in health: an agenda for action*. London: King's Fund, 1995.

209 Leather P, Morrison T. *The state of UK housing*. Bristol: The Policy Press, 1997.

210 Department of Trade and Industry. *Home and leisure accident research: twelfth annual report, 1988 data*. London: Department of Trade and Industry, Consumer Safety Unit, 1991.

211 Burridge R, Ormandy D, eds. *Unhealthy housing: research, remedies and reform*. London: E. and F.N. Spon, 1993.

212 Arblaster L, Hawtin M. *Health, housing and social policy*. London: Socialist Health Association, 1993.

213 Platt S, Martin C, Hunt S, Lewis C. Damp housing, mould growth and symptomatic health state. *British Medical Journal* 1989;**298**:1673–8.

214 Strachan D. Damp housing and childhood asthma: validation of reporting of symptoms. *British Medical Journal* 1988;**297**:1223–6.

215 Christopherson O. Mortality during the 1996/7 winter. *Population Trends* 1997;**90**:11–17.

216 Barnes C. *Disabled people in Britain and discrimination*. London: Hurst and Co., in association with the British Council of Organisations of Disabled People, 1991.

217 Palfreyman T. *Designing for accessibility: an introductory guide*. London: Centre for Accessible Environments, 1993.

218 Harris J, Sapey B, Stewart J. *Wheelchair housing and the estimation of need*. Preston: University of Central Lancashire, 1997.

219 Towner E, Dowswell T, Simpson G, Jarvis S. *Health promotion in childhood and young adolescence for the prevention of unintentional injuries*. London: Health Education Authority, 1996.

220 Mirrlees-Black C, Mayhew P, Percy A. *The 1996 British Crime Survey, England and Wales*. London: Government Statistical Office, 1996.

221 Mayhew P, Aye Maung N. *Surveying crime: findings from the 1992 British Crime Survey, no. 2/92.3*. London: Home Office, 1993.

222 Aye Maung N, Mirrlees-Black C. *Racially motivated crime: a British Crime Survey analysis*. London: Home Office Research and Planning Unit, 1994.

223 Kennedy B, Kawachi I, Prothrow-Stith D. Income distribution and mortality: cross-sectional ecological study of the Robin Hood index in the US. *British Medical Journal* 1996;**312**:1004–1007.

224 Kennedy B, Kawachi I, Prothrow-Stith D, Lochner K, Gupta V. Social capital, income inequality and firearm violent crime. *Social Science and Medicine* 1998;**47**:7–17.

225 Kawachi I, Kennedy B, Lochner K, Prothrow-Stith D. Social capital, income inequality and mortality. *American Journal of Public Health* 1997;**87**:1491–1498.

226 Wilkinson R. *Unhealthy societies: the afflictions of inequality*. London: Routledge, 1996.

227 Farrington D. *Understanding and preventing youth crime*. York: Joseph Rowntree Foundation, 1996.

228 Home Office Crime Prevention College and Home Office Crime Prevention Agency. *What works in crime prevention? Conference report*. London: Home Office Crime Prevention College, 1998.

229 Davis A. Submission to the Independent Inquiry into Inequalities in Health. Input paper: Transport and pollution. 1998.

230 Power A. Area-based poverty and resident empowerment. *Urban Studies* 1996;**33**:1535–1564.

231 Ong P, Blumenberg E. Job access, commute and travel burden among welfare recipients. *Urban Studies* 1998;**35**:77–93.

232 Piachaud D, Webb J. *The price of food: missing out on mass consumption.* London: Suntory and Toyota International Centre for Economics and Related Disciplines, 1996.

233 Watt I, Franks A, Sheldon T. Health and health care of rural populations in the UK: is it better or worse? *Journal of Epidemiology and Community Health* 1994;**48**:16–21.

234 Klaeboe R. *Measuring the environmental impact of road traffic in town areas: paper to Planning, Transport, Research and Computation Summer Annual Meeting.* London: Planning, Transport, Research and Computation, 1992.

235 Gillies P. Social capital: recognising the value of society. *Healthlines* 1997;**September**:15–17.

236 Department of Transport. *National travel survey, 1992–94.* London: HMSO, 1995.

237 Nicholl J, Freeman M, Williams B. Effects of subsidising bus travel on the occurrence of road traffic casualties. *Journal of Epidemiology and Community Health* 1987;**41**:50–54.

238 Sheffield City Council. *The bus booklet.* Sheffield: Sheffield City Council, 1986.

239 Goodwin P. *Subsidised public transport and the demand for travel: the South Yorkshire example.* Aldersot: Gower, 1983.

240 Rural Development Commission. *1997 survey of rural services.* Salisbury: Rural Development Commission, 1998.

241 Roberts I, Power C. Does the decline in child injury death rates vary by social class? *British Medical Journal* 1996;**313**:784–6.

242 Roberts I, Norton R, Taua B. Socioeconomic and ethnic differences in child pedestrian injury: the importance of exposure to risk. *Journal of Epidemiology and Community Health* 1996;**50**:162–165.

243 House of Commons. *Transport committee third report: risk reduction for vulnerable road users.* London: HMSO, 1996.

244 Davis A, Osborne P. *Safe routes to schools.* London: European Transport Forum, 1996.

245 NHS Centre for Reviews and Dissemination. Unintentional injuries in young people. *Effective Health Care* 1996;**2**.

246 Royal Commission on Environmental Pollution. *Transport and the environment: developments since 1994.* London: The Stationery Office, 1997.

247 Hedley S, Beevers S, Carslaw D, Lonsdale J. *Report on stage III of London air quality review: testing draft guidance on reviewing and assessing air quality.* Tunbridge Wells: South East Institute of Public Health, 1998.

248 London Research Centre. *Atmospheric emissions inventories for four urban areas.* London: Department of the Environment, Transport and the Regions, 1997.

249 Quality of Urban Air Review Group. *Urban air quality in the United Kingdom.* London: Department of the Environment, Transport and the Regions, 1993.

250 Department of Health Committee on the Medical Effects of Air Pollutants. *Quantification of the effects of air pollution on health in the United Kingdom.* London: The Stationery Office, 1998.

251 Department of Transport. *National road traffic forecasts (Great Britain).* London: HMSO, 1989.

252 Balarajan R. Ethnicity and variations in the nation's health. *Health Trends* 1995;**27**:114–119.

253 Department of Health. *Public health common data set: data files and definition.* Guildford: University of Surrey, National Institute of Epidemiology, 1997.

254 Department of the Environment, Transport and the Regions. *Road safety strategy: current problems and future solutions.* London: Department of the Environment, Transport and the Regions, 1997.

255 Department of the Environment, Transport and the Regions. *Vehicle speeds in Great Britain 1996. Statistical Bulletin (97)11.* London: Department of the Environment, Transport and the Regions, 1997.

256 Department of Transport. *Traffic calming: traffic and vehicle noise.* London: Department of Transport, 1996.

257 Wheway R, Millward A. *Child's play: facilitating play on housing estates.* Coventry: Chartered Institute of Housing/Joseph Rowntree Foundation, 1997.

258 Department of the Environment, Transport and the Regions. *Bus data: 1998 edition. A compendium of bus, coach and taxi statistics. Statistics Bulletin.* London: Department of the Environment, Transport and the Regions, 1998.

259 Department of the Environment, Transport and the Regions. *National Travel Survey 1994/96.* London: The Stationery Office, 1997.

260 Office for National Statistics. *Conceptions in England and Wales 1996.* Titchfield: Office for National Statistics, 1998.

261 Lang T, Whitehead M. Background. In: Dahlgren G, Nordgren P, Whitehead M, eds. *Health impact assessment of the EU common agricultural policy (second edition).* Stockholm: Swedish National Institute of Public Health, 1997.

262 European Union. *European Union budget 1998.* Luxembourg: European Union Publications Office, 1998.

263 Lang T. Time to reform the Common Agricultural Policy on health grounds? *Eurohealth* 1998;**4**:1–3.

264 Committee on Medical Aspects of Food Policy. *Report on health and social subjects no. 46: nutritional aspects of cardiovascular disease.* London: HMSO, 1994.

265 World Cancer Research Fund/American Cancer Research Fund. *Food, nutrition and the prevention of cancer.* Washington: World Cancer Research Fund/American Institute for Cancer Research, 1997.

266 Cadogan J, Eastell R, Jones N, Barker M. Milk intake and bone mineral acquisition in adolescent girls: randomised, controlled intervention trial. *British Medical Journal* 1997;**315**:1255–60.

267 Suleiman S, Nelson M, Li F, Buxton-Thomas M, Moniz C. Effect of calcium intake and physical activity level on bone mass and turnover in healthy, white, postmenopausal women. *American Journal of Clinical Nutrition* 1997;**66**:937–43.

268 Prentice A. Is nutrition important in osteoporosis? *Proceedings of the Nutrition Society* 1997;**56**:357–367.

269 Committee on Medical Aspects of Food Policy. *Report on health and social subjects no.41: dietary reference values for food energy and nutrients for the United Kingdom.* London: HMSO, 1991.

270 Pryer J, Vrijheid M, Nichols R, Elliott P. Who are the 'low energy reporters' in the Dietary and Nutritional Survey of British Adults. *Proceedings of the Nutrition Society* 1994;**53**:235A.

271 Ravelli A, van der Meulen J, Michels R, et al. Glucose tolerance in adults after prenatal exposure to the Dutch famine. *Lancet* 1998;**351**:173–177.

272 Clark P, Allen C, Law C, Shiell A, Godfrey K, Barker D. Weight gain in pregnancy, triceps skinfold thickness and blood pressure in the offspring. *Obstetrics and Gynecology* 1998;**91**:103–7.

273 Godfrey K, Forrester T, Barker D, et al. Maternal nutritional status in pregnancy and blood pressure in childhood. *British Journal of Obstetrics Gynaecology* 1994;**101**:398–403.

274 Forsen T, Eriksson J, Tuomilehto J, Teramo K, Osmond C, Barker D. Mother's weight in pregnancy and coronary heart disease in a cohort of Finnish men: follow up study. *British Medical Journal* 1997;**315**:837–840.

275 Campbell D, Hall M, Barker D, Cross J, Shiell A, Godfrey K. Diet in pregnancy and the offspring's blood pressure 40 years later. *British Journal of Obstetrics Gynaecology* 1996;**103**:273–280.

276 James W, Nelson M, Ralph A, Leather S. The contribution of nutrition to inequalities in health. *British Medical Journal* 1997;**314**:1545–9.

277 Marmot M, Shipley M, Rose G. Inequalities in death: specific explanations of a general pattern? *Lancet* 1984;**1**:1003–1006.

278 King J. *Family spending 1996–97.* London: The Stationery Office, 1997.

279 NCH Action for Children. *NCH poverty and nutrition survey (1991).* London: NCH, 1991.

280 Owens B. *Out of the frying pan.* London: Save the Children Foundation, 1997.

281 Mooney C. *Cost, availability and choice of healthy foods in some Camden supermarkets.* London: Hampstead Health Authority, 1987.

282 Department of Transport. *Transport statistics Great Britain, 1994.* London: HMSO, 1995.

283 Speak S, Cameron S, Woods R, Gilroy R. *Young single mothers: barriers to independent living.* London: Family Policy Studies Centre, 1995.

284 Leather S, Lobstein T. *Food and low income: a practical guide for advisors and supporters working with families and young people on low incomes.* London: National Food Alliance, 1994.

285 Raven H, Lang T, Dumonteil C. *Off our trolleys? Food retailing and the hypermarket economy.* London: Institute for Public Policy Research, 1995.

286 Sheiham A, Marmot M, Rawson D, Ruck N. Food values: health and diet. In: Jowell R, Witherspoon S, Brook L, eds. *British social attitudes: the 1987 report.* Aldershot: Ashgate Publishing Group, 1987.

287 Sheiham A, Marmot M, Taylor B, Brown A. Recipes for health. In: Jowell R, Witherspoon S, Brook L, eds. *British social attitudes: the 7th report.* Aldershot: Ashgate Publishing Group, 1990.

288 Graudal N, Galloe A, Garred P. Effects of sodium restriction on blood pressure, renin, aldosterone, catecholamines, cholesterols, and triglyceride. *Journal of the American Medical Association* 1998;**279**:1383–1391.

289 Daycare Trust. *Closing the childcare gap – partnerships for action: briefing paper 5.* London: Daycare Trust, 1997.

290 Daycare Trust. *A quality act? Developing a quality framework for childcare and pre-school services: briefing paper 3.* London: Daycare Trust, 1997.

291 Daycare Trust. *The childcare gap: briefing paper 1.* London: Daycare Trust, 1997.

292 Duncan A, Giles C. Should we subsidise pre-school child-care, and if so, how? *Fiscal Studies* 1996;**17**:39–61.

293 The Scottish Low Birthweight Study Group. The Scottish Low Birthweight Study 1: survival, growth, neuromotor and sensory impairment. *Archives of Disease in Childhood* 1992;**67**:675–681.

294 Vik T, Vatten L, Markestad T, Ahlsten G, Jacobsen G, Bakketeig L. Morbidity during the first year of life in small for gestational age infants. *Archives of Disease in Childhood* 1996;**75**:F33–F37.

295 Hack M, Weissman B, Breslau N, Klein N, Borawski-Clark E, Fanaroff A. Health of very low birthweight children during their first eight years. *Journal of Pediatrics* 1993;**122**:887–892.

296 Middle C, Johnson A, Alderdice F, Petty T, Macfarlane A. Birthweight and health and development at the age of 7 years. *Childcare, Health and Development* 1996;**22**:55–71.

297 Mutch L, Ashurst H, Macfarlane A. Birth weight and hospital admission before the age of 2 years. *Archives of Disease in Childhood* 1992;**67**:900–904.

298 Law C, Barker D, Richardson W, et al. Thinness at birth in a northern industrial town. *Journal of Epidemiology and Community Health* 1993;**47**:255–259.

299 Bourchard C, Bray G. *Regulation of body weight.* Chichester: John Wiley, 1996.

300 Duran-Tauleria E, Rona R, Chinn S. Factors associated with weight for height and skinfold thickness in British children. *Journal of Epidemiology and Community Health* 1995;**49**:466–473.

301 Hales C, Barker D, Clark P, et al. Fetal and infant growth and impaired glucose tolerance at age 64. *British Medical Journal* 1991;**303**:1019–1022.

302 Lithell H, McKeigue P, Berglund L, Mohsen R, Lithell U, Leon D. Relation of size at birth to non-insulin dependent diabetes and insulin concentrations in men aged 50–60 years. *British Medical Journal* 1996;**312**:406–410.

303 Leon D, Koupilova I, Lithell H, et al. Failure to realise growth potential in utero and adult obesity in relation to blood pressure in 50 year old Swedish men. *British Medical Journal* 1996;**312**:401–406.

304 Frankel S, Elwood P, Sweetnam P, Yarnell J, Davey Smith G. Birthweight, body-mass index in middle age, and incident coronary heart disease. *Lancet* 1996;**348**:1478–1480.

305 American Academy of Pediatrics, Working Group on Breastfeeding. Breastfeeding and the use of human milk. *Pediatrics* 1997;**100**:1035–39.

306 Hodnett E. Support from caregivers during childbirth. In: The Cochrane Database of Systematic Reviews, ed. *The Cochrane Library, Issue 2, 1998*. Oxford: Update Software (updated quarterly), 1998.

307 Renfrew M, Lang S. Breastfeeding technique. In: The Cochrane Database of Systematic Reviews, ed. *The Cochrane Library, Issue 2, 1998*. Oxford: Update Software (updated quarterly), 1998.

308 Kistin N, Abramson R, Dublin P. Effect of peer counsellors on breastfeeding initiation, exclusivity, and duration among low-income urban women. *Journal of Human Lactation* 1994;**10**:11–15.

309 Rossiter J. The effect of a culture-specific education program to promote breastfeeding among Vietnamese women in Sydney. *International Journal of Nursing Studies* 1994;**31**:369–9.

310 Hinds K, Gregory J. *National Diet and Nutrition Survey: Children aged 1¹/₂ to 4¹/₂ years. Volume 2: Report of the dental survey*. London: HMSO, 1995.

311 O'Brien M. *Children's dental health in the United Kingdom 1993*. London: HMSO, 1994.

312 Department of Health. *Public health common data set*. London: The Stationery Office, 1997.

313 Slade G, Spencer A, Davies M, Stewart J. Influence of exposure to fluoridated water on socioeconomic inequalities in children's caries exposure. *Community Dentistry and Oral Epidemiology* 1996;**24**:89–100.

314 Carmichael C, French A, Rugg-Gunn A, Ferrell R. The relationship between fluoridation, social class and caries experience in 5 year old children in Newcastle and Northumberland in 1987. *British Dental Journal* 1989;**167**:57–61.

315 Jones C, Taylor G, Whittle J, Evans D, Trotter D. Water fluoridation, tooth decay in 5 year olds, and social deprivation measured by the Jarman score: analysis of data from British dental surveys. *British Medical Journal* 1997;**315**:514–7.

316 Blair P, Fleming P, Bensley D, et al. Smoking and the sudden infant death syndrome: results from 1993–5 case-control study for Confidential Enquiry into Stillbirths and Deaths in Infancy. *British Medical Journal* 1996;**313**:195–198.

317 Chollat-Traquet C. *Women and tobacco*. Geneva: World Health Organisation, 1992.

318 Faculty of Public Health Medicine Committee on Health Promotion. *Women and smoking: health promotion report no 39*. London: Royal College of Physicians, Faculty of Public Health Medicine, 1995.

319 Royal College of Physicians. *A report of a working party on smoking in the young*. London: Royal College of Physicians, 1992.

320 Department of Health. *Report of the Scientific Committee on Tobacco and Health*. London: The Stationery Office, 1998.

321 Fogelman K, Manor O. Smoking in pregnancy and development into early adulthood. *British Medical Journal* 1988;**297**:1233–1236.

322 Health Education Authority. *Smoking and pregnancy: guidance for purchasers and providers*. London: Health Education Authority, 1994.

323 Arblaster L, Entwistle V, Fullerton D, et al. *A review of the effectiveness of health promotion interventions aimed at reducing inequalities in health*. York: NHS Centre for Reviews and Dissemination, 1998.

324 Lumley J. Strategies for reducing smoking in pregnancy. In: The Cochrane Database of Systematic Reviews, ed. *The Cochrane Library, Issue 2, 1995*. Oxford: Update Software, 1995.

325 Batten L. *Low income, smoking, pregnancy and the transtheoretical model*. Southampton: University of Southampton, Department of Psychology, 1997.

326 Graham H. *When life's a drag: women, smoking and disadvantage*. London: HMSO, 1993.

327 Dorsett R, Marsh A. *The health trap: poverty, smoking and lone parenthood*. London: Policy Studies Institute, 1998.

328 Home Office, Department of Health, Department for Education and Employment, Welsh Office. *Working together under the Children's Act 1989*. London: HMSO, 1991.

329 Leiter J, Meyers K, Zingraff M. Substantiated and unsubstantiated cases of child maltreatment: do their consequences differ? *Social Work Research* 1994; **18**:67–82.

330 Department of Health. *Children looked-after by local authorities: year ending 31 March 1996.* London: Department of Health, 1997.

331 Creighton S. *Child abuse trends in England and Wales, 1988–1990.* London: National Society for the Prevention of Cruelty to Children, 1992.

332 Gillham B, Tanner G, Cheyne B, Freeman I, Rooney M, Lambie A. Unemployment rates, single parent density, and indices of child poverty: their relationship to different categories of child abuse and neglect. *Child Abuse and Neglect* 1998;**22**:79–90.

333 NCH Action for Children. *National children's homes, factfile 98.* London: NCH, 1997.

334 Roberts H. Children, inequalities, and health. *British Medical Journal* 1997;**314**:1122–1125.

335 Gibbons J, Thorpe S, Wilkinson P. *Family support and prevention: studies in local areas – purposes and organisation of preventive work with families.* London: HMSO, 1990.

336 Oakley A. *Social support and motherhood.* Oxford: Blackwell, 1992.

337 Hodnett E. Support from caregivers during at-risk pregnancy. In: The Cochrane Database of Systematic Reviews, ed. *The Cochrane Library, Issue 2, 1998.* Oxford: Update Software (updated quarterly), 1998.

338 Elbourne D, Oakley A, Chalmers I. Social and psychological support during pregnancy. In: Chalmers I, Enkin M, Keirse M, eds. *Effective Care in Pregnancy and Childbirth, vol.1.* Oxford: Oxford University Press, 1989.

339 Hodnett E, Roberts I. Home-based social support for socially disadvantaged mothers. In: The Cochrane Database of Systematic Reviews, ed. *The Cochrane Library, Issue 2, 1998.* Oxford: Update Software (updated quarterly), 1998.

340 Seeley S, Murray L, Cooper P. The outcome for mothers and babies of health visitor intervention. *Health Visitor* 1996;**69**:135–138.

341 Holden J, Sagovsky R, Cox J. Counselling in a general practice setting: a controlled study of health visitor intervention in the treatment of postnatal depression. *British Medical Journal* 1989;**298**:223–226.

342 Murray L. Postpartum depression and child development. *Psychological Medicine* 1997;**27**:253–260.

343 Barker W, Anderson R, Chalmers C. *Child protection: the impact of the child development programme (evaluation document 14).* Bristol: University of Bristol, Early Child Development Unit, 1994.

344 Barnardos. Submission to the Independent Inquiry into Inequalities in Health. 1997.

345 Barlow J. *Systematic review of the effectiveness of parent-training programmes in improving behaviour problems in children aged 3–10 years.* Oxford: University of Oxford, Health Services Research Unit, 1997.

346 Olds D, Eckenrode J, Henderson C, et al. Long-term effects of home visitation on maternal life course and child abuse and neglect. Fifteen-year follow-up of a randomized trial. *Journal of the American Medical Association* 1997;**278**:637–643.

347 Oakley A, Hickey O, Rajan L, Hickey A. Social support in pregnancy: does it have long term effects? *Journal of Reproductive Infant Psychology* 1996;**14**:7–22.

348 Baldwin N, Carruthers L. *Developing neighbourhood support and child protection strategies.* Aldershot: Ashgate, 1998.

349 Barker W, Anderson R. *The child development programme: an evaluation of process and outcomes (evaluation document 9).* Bristol: University of Bristol, Early Child Development Unit, 1988.

350 Robinson J. Submission to the Independent Inquiry into Inequalities in Health: Health Visiting. 1998.

351 Action on After Care Consortium. *Too much, too young.* London: Action on After Care Consortium, 1996.

352 Save the Children. *You're on your own.* London: Save the Children/Action on Aftercare Consortium, 1995.

353 Health Advisory Service Report. *Children and young people: substance misuse services.* London: The Stationery Office, 1996.

354 Buchanan A, Brinke J. *Outcomes from parenting experiences.* York: Joseph Rowntree Foundation, 1997.

355 Royal College of Paediatrics and Child Health. Submission to the Independent Inquiry into Inequalities in Health. 1997.

356 Soni Raleigh V. Suicide patterns and trends in people of Indian sub-continent and Caribbean origin in England and Wales. *Ethnicity and Health* 1996;**1**:55–63.

357 Charlton J, Dunnell K, Evans B, Jenkins R. Suicide deaths in England and Wales: trends in factors associated with suicide deaths. In: Jenkins R, Griffiths S, Wylie I, Hawton K, Morgan G, Tylee A, eds. *The prevention of suicide.* London: HMSO, 1994.

358 Spirito A, Brown L, Overholser J, Fritz G. Attempted suicide in adolescence: a review and critique of the literature. *Clinical Psychology Review* 1989;**9**:335–363.

359 Hawton K, Fagg J, Platts S, Hawkins M. Factors associated with suicide following parasuicide in young people. *British Medical Journal* 1993;**306**:1641–1644.

360 Marttunen M, Aro H, Lonnqvist J. Precipitant stressors in adolescent suicide. *Journal of the American Academy of Child and Adolescent Psychiatry* 1993;**32**:1178–1183.

361 Diekstra R, Kienhorst C, de Wilde E. Suicide and suicidal behaviour among adolescents. In: Rutter M, Smith DJ, eds. *Psychosocial disorders in young people: time trends and their causes.* Chichester: Wiley, 1995.

362 Appleby L. *National Confidential Inquiry into Suicide and Homicide by People with Mental Illness: progress report.* London: Department of Health, 1997.

363 NHS Centre for Reviews and Dissemination. Mental health promotion in high risk groups. *Effective Health Care* 1997;**3.**

364 Tyrer P, Coid J, Simmonds S, Joseph P, Marriott S. Community mental health team management for those with severe mental illnesses and disordered personality. In: The Cochrane Database of Systematic Reviews, ed. *The Cochrane Library, Issue 2, 1998.* Oxford: Update Software (updated quarterly), 1998.

365 World Health Organisation. *Ottawa Charter for Health Promotion.* Copenhagen: World Health Organisation, 1990.

366 Wellings K, Fields J, Johnson A, Wadsworth J. *Sexual behaviour in Britain: the national survey of sexual attitudes and lifestyle.* London: Penguin, 1994.

367 Health Education Authority. *Reducing the rate of teenage conceptions: towards a national programme.* London: Health Education Authority, 1998.

368 Chinn S, Rona R. Trends in weight-for-height and triceps skinfold thickness for English and Scottish children, 1972–1982 and 1982–1990. *Paediatric and Perinatal Epidemiology* 1994;**8**:90–106.

369 US Department of Health and Human Services. *Physical activity and health: a report of the Surgeon General.* Atlanta: US Department of Health and Human Services, Centers for Disease Control and Prevention, National Center for Chronic Disease Prevention and Health Promotion, 1996.

370 Berlin J, Colditz G. A meta-analysis of physical activity in the prevention of coronary heart disease. *American Journal of Epidemiology* 1990;**132**:639–646.

371 Happanen N, Miilunpalo S, Pasanen M, Oja P, Vuori I. Asssociation between leisure time physical activity and 10-year body mass change among working-aged men and women. *International Journal of Obesity* 1997;**21**:288–296.

372 Blair S, Connelly J. How much physical activity should we do: the case for moderate amounts and intensities of physical activity. *Research Quarterly for Exercise and Sport* 1996;**67**:193–205.

373 Pate R, Pratt M, Blair S, et al. Physical activity and public health: a recommendation from the Centers for Disease Control and Prevention and the American College of Sports Medicine. *Journal of the American Medical Association* 1995;**273**:402–407.

374 Hillsdon M, Thorogood M. A systematic review of exercise promotion strategies. *British Journal of Sports Medicine* 1996;**91**:2596–2604.

375 Jarvis M. Patterns and predictors of smoking cessation in the general population. In: Bolliger C, Fagerstrom K, eds. *Progress in respiratory research: the tobacco epidemic.* Basel: S Karger AG, 1997.

376 Peto R, Lopez A, Boreham J, Heath C, Then M. *Mortality from tobacco in developed countries, 1950–2000.* Oxford: Oxford University Press, 1994.

377   Callum C. *The UK smoking epidemic: deaths in 1995.* London: Health Education Authority, 1998.

378   Andrews R, Franke G. The determinations of cigarette consumption: a meta analysis. *Journal of Public Policy and Marketing* 1991;81–100.

379   Townsend J. *Price, tax and smoking in Europe.* Copenhagen: World Health Organisation, 1998.

380   Reid D. Tobacco control: overview. *British Medical Bulletin* 1996;**52**:108–120.

381   Lewit E, Coate D. The potential for using excise taxes to reduce smoking. *Journal of Health Economics* 1982;**1**:121–145.

382   Wasserman J, Manning W, Newhouse J, Winkler J. The effects of excise taxes and regulations on cigarette smoking. *Journal of Health Economics* 1991;**10**:43–64.

383   Townsend J, Roderick P, Cooper J. Cigarette smoking by socioeconomic group, sex and age: effects of price, income, and health publicity. *British Medical Journal* 1994;**309**:923–927.

384   Chaloupka F, Grossman M. *Price, tobacco control policies and youth smoking: working paper 5740.* Cambridge, MA: National Bureau of Economic Research, 1996.

385   Chaloupka F, Wechsler H. Price, tobacco control policies and smoking among young adults. *Journal of Health Economics* 1997;**16**:359–373.

386   Lewit E, Hyland A, Kerrebrock N, Cummings K. Price, public policy and smoking in young people. *Tobacco Control* 1997;**6**:S17–S25.

387   Fry V, Pashardes P. *Changing patterns of smoking: are there economic causes?* London: Institute for Fiscal Studies, 1998.

388   Marsh A, McKay S. *Poor smokers.* London: Policy Studies Institute, 1994.

389   Silagy C, Mant D, Fowler G, Lodge M. Meta-analysis on efficacy of nicotine replacement therapies in smoking cessation. *Lancet* 1994;**43**:139–142.

390   Tang J, Law M, Wald N. How effective is nicotine replacement therapy in helping people to stop smoking? *British Medical Journal* 1994;**308**:21–26.

391   Sonderskov J, Olsen J, Sabroe S, Meillier L, Overvad K. Nicotine patches in smoking cessation: a randomised trial among over-the-counter customers in Denmark. *American Journal of Epidemiology* 1997;**145**:309–318.

392   Pierce J, Gilpin E, Farkas A. Nicotine patch use in the general population: results from the 1993 California Tobacco Survey. *Journal of the National Cancer Institute* 1995;**87**:87–93.

393   Silagy C, Mant D, Fowler G, Lancaster T. Nicotine replacement therapy for smoking cessation. In: The Cochrane Database of Systematic Reviews, ed. *The Cochrane Library, Issue 2, 1998.* Oxford: Update Software (updated quarterly), 1998.

394   Fowler G. Nicotine replacement should be prescribable on the NHS. *British Medical Journal* 1997;**314**:1827.

395   Hughes J, Wadland W, Fenwick J, Lewis J, Bickel W. Effect of cost on the self-administration and efficacy of nicotine gum: a preliminary study. *Preventive Medicine* 1991;**20**:486–496.

396   Health Education Board for Scotland/Action on Smoking and Health. *A smoking cessation policy for Scotland.* Edinburgh: Health Education Board for Scotland/Action on Smoking and Health, 1998.

397   Drever F, Bunting J, Harding D. Male mortality from major causes of death. In: Drever F, Whitehead M, eds. *Health inequalities: decennial supplement: DS Series no.15.* London: The Stationery Office, 1997.

398   Forcier M. Unemployment and alcohol abuse: a review. *Journal of Occupational Medicine* 1988;**30**:246–251.

399   Hammarstroem A. Health consequences of youth unemployment: review from a gender perspective. *Social Science and Medicine* 1994;**38**:699–709.

400   Catalano R. The health effects of economic insecurity. *American Journal of Public Health* 1991;**81**:1148–1152.

401   Gill B, Meltzer H, Hinds K, Petticrew M. *Office of Population Censuses and Surveys: surveys of psychiatric morbidity in Great Britain: psychiatric morbidity among homeless people (report 7).* London: HMSO, 1996.

402 Hall W, Farrell M. Co-morbidity of mental disorders with substance misuse. *British Journal of Psychiatry* 1997;**171**:4–5.

403 Harrison L. *Alcohol problems in the community*. London: Routledge, 1996.

404 Colhoun H, Ben-Shlomo Y, Dong W, Marmot M. Ecological analysis of collectivity of alcohol consumption in England: importance of the average drinker. *British Medical Journal* 1997;**314**:1164–68.

405 Edwards G, Anderson P, Babor T, et al. *Alcohol policy and the public good*. New York: Oxford University Press, 1994.

406 Richardson J, Crowley S. Optimum alcohol taxation: balancing consumption and external costs. *Health Economics* 1994;**3**:73–87.

407 Ponicki W, Holder H, Gruenewald P, Romelsjo A. Altering alcohol price by ethanol content: results from a Swedish tax policy in 1992. *Addiction* 1997;**92**:859–70.

408 Marmot M. Inequality, deprivation and alcohol use. *Addiction* 1997;**Supplement 1**:S13–S20.

409 Sutton M, Godfrey C. A grouped data regression approach to estimating economic and social influences on individual drinking behaviour. *Health Economics* 1995;**4**:237–247.

410 British Medical Association. *Driving impairment through alcohol and other drugs*. London: British Medical Association, 1996.

411 Peacock C. International policies on alcohol-impaired driving: a review. *International Journal of Addiction* 1992;**27**:187–208.

412 Smith J, Harding S. Mortality of women and men using alternative social classifications. In: Drever F, Whitehead M, eds. *Health inequalities: decennial supplement: DS Series no.15.* London: The Stationery Office, 1997.

413 Drever F, Whitehead M. Mortality in regions and local authority districts in the 1990s: exploring the relationship with deprivation. *Population Trends* 1995;**82**:19–26.

414 Office of Population Censuses and Surveys. *Adult dental health survey 1988.* London: HMSO, 1990.

415 Martin J, White A. *Office of Population Censuses and Surveys: surveys of disability in Great Britain: report 2 – the financial circumstances of disabled adults living in private households.* London: HMSO, 1988.

416 Grindey S, Winyard S. *Losing sight of blindness*. London: RNIB, 1997.

417 Landes R, Popay J. "My sight is poor but I'm getting on now": the health and social care needs of older people with visual problems. *Health and Social Care* 1993;**1**:325–35.

418 Reinstein D, Dorward N, Wormald R, et al. Correctable undetected visual acuity deficit in patients aged 65 and over attending an accident and emergency department. *British Journal of Ophthalmology* 1993;**77**:293–6.

419 Webster E, Barnes G. Eye tests in the elderly: factors associated with attendance and diagnostic yield in non-attenders. *Journal of the Royal Society of Medicine* 1992;**85**:614–6.

420 Arber S, Ginn J. *Gender and later life: a sociological analysis of resources and constraints.* London: Sage, 1991.

421 Arber S, Ginn J. *Connecting gender and ageing: a sociological approach.* Buckingham: Open University Press, 1995.

422 NHS Centre for Reviews and Dissemination. Preventing falls and subsequent injury in older people. *Effective Health Care* 1996 **2**.

423 Hamilton K, Jenkins L, Gregory A. *Women and transport: bus deregulation in West Yorkshire.* Bradford: University of Bradford, 1991.

424 Gant R, Smith J. Journey patterns of the elderly and disabled in the Cotswolds: a spatial analysis. *Social Science and Medicine* 1988;**27**:173–190.

425 Martin J, White A, Meltzer H. *Office of Population Censuses and Surveys: surveys of disability in Great Britain: report 4 – disabled adults: services, transport and employment.* London: HMSO, 1989.

426 Hine J, Russell J. The impact of traffic on pedestrian behaviour: assessing the traffic barrier on radial routes. *Traffic Engineering and Control* 1996;**February**:81–85.

427 Langlois J, Keyl P, Guralnik J, Foley D, Marottoli R, Wallace R. Characteristics of older pedestrians who have difficulty crossing the street. *American Journal of Public Health* 1997;**87**:393–397.

428 Khaw K. Submission to the Independent Inquiry into Inequalities in Health. Input paper: Older people. 1997.

429 Chaturvedi N, Ben-Shlomo Y. From the surgery to the surgeon: does deprivation influence consultation and operation rates? *British Journal of General Practice* 1995;**45**:127–131.

430 Jones H, Yates J, Spurgeon P, Fielder A. Geographical variations in rates of ophthalmic surgery. *British Journal of Ophthalmology* 1996;**80**:784–788.

431 Wormald R, Wright L, Courtney P, Beaumont B, Haines A. Visual problems in the elderly population and implications for services. *British Medical Journal* 1992;**304**:1226.

432 Grimley-Evans J. Submission to the Independent Inquiry into Inequalities in Health: Ageism. 1998.

433 Barot R. *The racism problematic: contemporary sociological debates on race and ethnicity.* Lewiston: The Edwin Mellen Press, 1996.

434 Owen D. *Ethnic minorities in Great Britain: settlement patterns, national ethnic minority data archive 1991 – census statistical paper no.1.* Warwick: University of Warwick, Centre for Research in Ethnic Relations, 1992.

435 Commission for Racial Equality. *The Irish in Britain.* London: Commission for Racial Equality, 1997.

436 Owen D. Spatial variations in ethnic minority groups populations in Great Britain. *Population Trends* 1994;**78**:23–33.

437 Owen D. *Ethnic minorities in Great Britain: age and gender structure, national ethnic minority data archive 1991 – census statistical paper no.2.* Warwick: University of Warwick, Centre for Research in Ethnic Relations, 1993.

438 Coleman D, Salt J. *Ethnicity in the 1991 Census: volume 1, demographic characteristics of the ethnic minority populations.* London: HMSO, 1996.

439 Harding S, Maxwell R. Differences in the mortality of migrants. In: Drever F, Whitehead M, eds. *Health inequalities: decennial supplement: DS Series no.15.* London: The Stationery Office, 1997.

440 Balarajan R, Soni Raleigh V. *Ethnicity and health in England.* London: HMSO, 1995.

441 Nazroo J. *The health of Britain's ethnic minorities: findings from a national survey.* London: Policy Studies Institute, 1997.

442 McKeigue P, Sevak L. *Coronary heart disease in South Asian communities.* London: Health Education Authority, 1994.

443 De Cock K, Low N. HIV and AIDS, other sexually transmitted diseases, and tuberculosis in ethnic minorities in United Kingdom: is surveillance serving its purpose? *British Medical Journal* 1997;**314**:1747–31.

444 Owen D. *Irish-born people in Great Britain: settlement patterns and socio-economic circumstances. Census statistical paper no.9.* Warwick: University of Warwick, Centre for Research in Ethnic Relations, 1995.

445 Cochrane R, Bal S. Mental hospital admission rates of immigrants to England: a comparison of 1971 and 1981. *Social Psychiatry and Psychiatric Epidemiology* 1989;**24**:2–11.

446 Health Education Authority. *Guidelines: promoting physical activity with black and minority ethnic groups.* London: Health Education Authority, 1997.

447 Marmot M, Adelstein A, Bulusu L. *Immigrant mortality in England and Wales 1970–78: causes of death by country of birth.* London: HMSO, 1984.

448 Bhopal RS, Donaldson LJ. Health education for ethnic minorities: current provision and future directions. *Health Education Journal* 1988;**47**:137–140.

449 Bhopal R. Is research into ethnicity and health racist, unsound, or important science? *British Medical Journal* 1997;**314**:1751–1756.

450 Block A. *Access to benefits: the information needs of ethnic minorities.* London: Policy Studies Institute, 1993.

451 Law I, Hylton C, Karmani A, Deacon A. *Racial equality and social security service delivery.* Leeds: University of Leeds, 1994.

452 Berthoud R. *Social security and race: an agenda. Policy Studies Institute working paper.* London: Policy Studies Institute, 1987.

453 Bowes A, Dar N, Sim D. *Too white, too rough and too many problems: a study of Pakistani housing in Britain.* Stirling: University of Stirling, 1997.

454 Gardiner C, Hill R. Analysis of access to cars from the 1991 UK Census Samples of Anonymised Records: a case study of the elderly population of Sheffield. *Urban Studies* 1996;**33**:269–281.

455 Jones L. Putting transport on the social policy agenda. In: May M, Brinsdon E, Craig G, eds. *Social policy review 8.* London: Longmans, 1997.

456 Lawson S, Edwards P. The involvement of ethnic minorities in road accidents: data from three studies of young pedestrian casualties. *Traffic Engineering and Control* 1991;**January**:12–19.

457 Rudat K. *Black and minority ethnic groups in England: health and lifestyles.* London: Health Education Authority, 1994.

458 Smaje C, Le grand J. Ethnicity, equity and the use of health services in the British National Health Service. *Social Science and Medicine* 1997;**45**:485–96.

459 Lear J, Lawrence I, Pohl J, Burden A. Myocardial infarction and thrombolysis: a comparison of the Indian and European populations on a coronary care unit. *Journal of the Royal College of Physicians* 1994;**28**:143–147.

460 Lear J, Lawrence I, Burden A, Pohl J. A comparison of stress test referral rates and outcome between Asians and Europeans. *Journal of the Royal Society of Medicine* 1994;**87**:661–662.

461 Nazroo J. *Ethnicity and mental health: findings from a national community survey.* London: Policy Studies Institute, 1997.

462 Naish J, Brown J, Denton B. Intercultural consultations: investigation of factors that deter non-English speaking women from attending their general practitioners for cervical screening. *British Medical Journal* 1994;**309**:1126–8.

463 Bhopal R, White M. Health promotion for ethnic minorities: past, present and future. In: Ahmad W, ed. *'Race' and health in contemporary Britain.* Buckingham: Open University Press, 1993.

464 Macintyre S, Maciver S, Soomans A. Area, class and health: should we be focusing on places or people? *Journal of Social Policy* 1993 **22**:213–234.

465 Sloggett A, Joshi H. Higher mortality in deprived areas: community or personal disadvantage. *British Medical Journal* 1994 **309**:1470–74.

466 Halpern D. Minorities and mental health. *Social Science and Medicine* 1993 **36**:597–607.

467 Smaje C. Ethnic residential concentration and health: evidence for a positive effect? *Policy and Politics* 1995 **23**:251–69.

468 Begum N. *Something to be proud of... the lives of Asian disabled people in Waltham Forest.* London: Waltham Forest Race Relations Unit, 1992.

469 Tickle L. Mortality trends in the United Kingdom, 1982 to 1992. *Population Trends* 1996;**86**:21–28.

470 Dunnell K. Deaths among 15–44 year olds. *Population Trends* 1991;**64**:38–43.

471 Soni Raleigh V, Kiri V. Life expectancy in England: variations and trends by gender, health authority, and level of deprivation. *Journal of Epidemiology and Community Health* 1997;**51**:649–658.

472 Macintyre S, Hunt K. Socio-economic postion, gender and health. *Journal of Health Psychology* 1997;**2**:315–334.

473 Nathanson C. Sex, illness and medical care: a review of data, theory and method. *Social Science and Medicine* 1977;**11**:13–25.

474 Arber S. Submission to the Independent Inquiry into Inequalities in Health. Input paper: Gender. 1997.

475 Macintyre S, Hunt K, Sweeting H. Gender differences in health: are things really as simple as they seem? *Social Science and Medicine* 1996;**42**:617–624.

476 Sweeting H. Reversals of fortune? Sex differences in health in childhood and adolescence. *Social Science and Medicine* 1994;**40**:77–90.

477 Macran S, Clark L, Joshi H. Women's health: dimensions and differentials. *Social Science and Medicine* 1996;**42**:1203–16.

478 Cooper C, Melton L. Magnitude and impact of osteoporosis and fractures. In: Marcus R, Feldman D, Kelsey J, eds. *Osteoporosis*. San Diego: Academic Press, 1996.

479 Martin J, Meltzer H, Elliot D. *The prevalence of disability among adults: report 1*. London: HMSO, 1988.

480 Office of Population Censuses and Surveys. *Living in Britain: results from the general household survey 1994*. London: HMSO, 1996.

481 Office of Population Censuses and Surveys. *1991 Census: communal establishments*. London: HMSO, 1993.

482 Wardle J, Farrell M, Hillsdon M, Jarvis M, Sutton S, Thorogood M. Submission to the Independent Inquiry into Inequalities in Health. Input paper: Health-related behaviours. 1997.

483 Balding J. *Young people in 1996*. Exeter: School Health Education Unit, 1997.

484 Power C. Health related behaviour. In: Botting B, ed. *The health of our children, decennial supplement: the Registrar General's decennial supplement for England and Wales*. London: HMSO, 1995.

485 Central Statistical Office. *Labour force survey quarterly bulletin (No.14)*. London: HMSO, 1995.

486 Department of Employment. *New earnings survey 1995*. London: HMSO, 1995.

487 Kiernan K. Men and women at work and at home. In: Jowell R, Witherspoon S, Brook L, eds. *British Social Attitudes: the 8th Report*. Aldershot: Ashgate Publishing Group, 1991.

488 Corti L, Dex S. Informal carers and employment. *Employment Gazette* 1995;**103**:101–107.

489 Lister R. *Women's economic dependency and social security*. Manchester: Equal Opportunities Commission, 1992.

490 Bynner J, Ferri E, Shepherd P, eds. *Twenty-something in the 1990s: getting on, getting by, getting nowhere*. Aldershot: Ashgate, 1997.

491 Elliot J, Huppert F. In sickness and in health: associations between physical and mental well-being, employment and parental status in a British nationwide sample of married women. *Psychological Medicine* 1991;**21**:515–24.

492 Baker D, Taylor H. Inequality in health and health service use for mothers of young children in south west England. *Journal of Epidemiology and Community Health* 1997;**51**:74–79.

493 Atkins S. *Critical paths: designing for secure travel*. London: Design Council, 1989.

494 Arber S, Ginn J. Women and ageing. *Reviews in Clinical Gerontology* 1994;**4**:93–102.

495 Ross J. *The National Health Service in Great Britain*. Oxford: Oxford University Press, 1952.

496 Goddard M, Smith P. *Equity of access to health care*. York: University of York, 1998.

497 Expert Advisory Group on Cancer. *A policy framework for commissioning cancer services*. London: Department of Health, 1995.

498 Carr-Hill R, Place M, Posnett J. Access and utilisation of health care services. In: Sheldon T, Posnett J, eds. *Concentration and Choice in Healthcare*. London: Financial Times Healthcare, 1997.

499 Benzeval M, Judge K. Access to healthcare in England: continuing inequalities in the distribution of general practitioners. *Journal of Public Health Medicine* 1996;**18**:33–40.

500 Birmingham Health Authority. *Birmingham annual public health report: closing the gap*. Birmingham: Birmingham Health Authority, 1995.

501 East London and The City Health Authority. *Annual public health report 1997/98: health in the East End*. London: East London and The City Health Authority, 1998.

502 Flynn P, Knight D. *Inequalities in health in the North West*. Warrington: NHS Executive, North West, 1998.

503 Bardsley M, Bevan P, Gill M, Jacobson B. *Health in the capital: a city-wide perspective*. London: The Health of Londoner's Project, 1997.

504 Chenet L, McKee M. Challenges of monitoring use of secondary care at local level: a study based in London, UK. *Journal of Epidemiology and Community Health* 1996;**50**:359–365.

505 Slack R, Ferguson B, Ryder S. Analysis of hospitalisation rates by electoral ward: relationship to accessibility and deprivation data. *Health Services Management Research* 1996;**10**:24–31.

506 Watson J, Cowen P, Lewis R. The relationship between asthma and admission rates, routes of admission and socioeconomic deprivation. *European Respiratory Journal* 1996;**9**:2087–2093.

507 McCormick A, Fleming D, Charlton J. *Morbidity statistics from general practice fourth national study 1991–92*. London: The Stationery Office, 1995.

508 NHS Executive. *Clinical efectiveness indicators: a consultation document*. Leeds: NHS Executive, 1998.

509 Lakhani A. Submission to the Independent Inquiry into Inequalities in Health: Health outcomes. 1998.

510 Gillam S, Jarman B, White P, Law R. Ethnic differences in consultation rates in urban general practice. *British Medical Journal* 1989;**299**:953–957.

511 King's Fund. *London's mental health: the report to the King's Fund London Commission*. London: King's Fund, 1997.

512 Mays N. Geographical resource allocation in the English National Health Service, 1971–1994: the tension between normative and empirical approaches. *International Journal of Epidemiology* 1995;**24**:S96–S102.

513 Sheldon T. Formula fever: allocating resources in the NHS. *British Medical Journal* 1997;**315**:964.

514 Parsons L, Day S. Improving obstetric outcomes in ethnic minorities: an evaluation of health advocacy in Hackney. *Journal of Public Health Medicine* 1992;**14**:183–191.

515 Judge K, Mays N. Allocating resources for health and social care in England. *British Medical Journal* 1994;**308**:1363–6.

516 Medical Practices Committee. *Newsletter 3 July*. London: Medical Practices Committee, 1997.

517 Boyle S, Hamblin R. *The health economy of London: a report to the King's Fund London Commission*. London: King's Fund, 1997.

518 Johnstone F, Lucy J, Scott-Samuel A, Whitehead M. *Deprivation and health in North Cheshire: an equity audit of health services*. Liverpool: Liverpool Public Health Observatory, 1996.

519 London Strategic Review Independent Advisory Panel. *Health services in London: a strategic review (the Turnberg Report)*. London: Department of Health, 1997.

520 Hirst M, Lunt N, Atkin K. Were practice nurses equitably distributed across England and Wales 1988–1995? *Journal of Health Services Research and Policy* 1998;**3**:31–38.

521 Worrall A, Rea J, Ben-Shlomo Y. Counting the cost of social disadvantage in primary care: retrospective analysis of patient data. *British Medical Journal* 1997;**314**:38–42.

522 NHS Executive. *Annual report: the four Rs, recruitment, retention, refreshment and reflection*. Leeds: NHS Executive, 1997.

523 NHS Executive. *1998/1999 Health Authority Revenue Cash Limits Exposition Book*. Leeds: NHS Executive, 1997.

524 NHS Executive. *HIV/AIDS funding: EL(97)18*. Leeds: NHS Executive, 1997.

525 Laing W. *Laing's review of private healthcare*. London: Laing and Buisson, 1997.

526 Clinical Standards Advisory Group. *Access to and availability of coronary artery bypass graft (CABG) and coronary angioplasty. Report of a Clinical Standards Advisory Group Working Group*. London: HMSO, 1993.

527 Black N, Langham S, Coshall C, Parker J. Impact of the 1991 NHS reforms on the availability and use of coronary revascularisation in the UK (1987–1995). *Heart* 1996;**72**.

528 Liverpool City Council, Liverpool Health Authority. *Liverpool Healthy City 2000*. Liverpool: Liverpool City Council/Liverpool Health Authority, 1996.

529 Department of Health. *Chief Medical Officer's project to strengthen the public health function: report of emerging findings*. London: Department of Health, 1998.

ANNEXES

A. Letter from the Minister for Public Health

B. Process of the Inquiry

C. Acknowledgements

D. Papers, Submissions and Evidence to the Inquiry

Letter from the Minister for Public Health

Sir Donald Acheson
International Centre for Health & Society
University College, London
1–19 Torrington Place
LONDON WC1 6BT

10 July 1997

Review of inequalities in health

I thought it might be helpful to follow up our most useful conversation last Friday in order to confirm both where we had got to and the outstanding action on which you agreed to come back to me.

We have now agreed slightly revised terms of reference as follows:

"1. To moderate a Department of Health review of the latest available information on inequalities of health, using data from the Office for National Statistics, the Department of Health and elsewhere. The data review would summarise the evidence of inequalities of health and expectation of life in England and identify trends.

2. In the light of that evidence, to conduct – within the broad framework of the Government's overall financial strategy – an independent review to identify priority areas for future policy development, which scientific and expert evidence indicates are likely to offer opportunities for Government to develop beneficial, cost effective and affordable interventions to reduce health inequalities.

3. The review will report to the Secretary of State for Health. The report will be published and its conclusions, based on evidence, will contribute to the development of a new strategy for health."

We discussed the timing of your report. You were very concerned that a credible and reputable piece of work covering such a broad spectrum of issues could not be completed by January 1998 as we had originally hoped. However, you undertook to produce that part of your report which related to the work of the NHS by January 1998. You will then seek to produce by the end of March 1998 such further work as you are able to do properly in the time available. Any outstanding sections would form part of the final report to be delivered by the end of June.

However, proceeding on that basis makes it all the more important that the Department, whether through the CMO or the Secretariat, are kept in very close touch with your emerging findings so that these can be taken into account in the drafting of the Health Strategy White Paper which I intend to publish in the middle of next year. As I said, I recognise the time pressure which my overall timetable imposes on you but I do think it is vital to ensure that your work is relevant to the development of my new strategy for health.

Finally, we discussed the size and composition of the group of experts who you would like to assist you. As I said, I am concerned that the current proposals would create too large and unmanageable a group and you kindly undertook to consider how to reduce its size whilst covering all the major interests. I am most grateful to you for agreeing to consider these points further and to come back to me in due course. On further reflection, given the scientific basis of the evidence you intend to produce, scientists are clearly your essential resource for further advice.

The Secretary of State and I are both delighted that you and I have now been able to reach agreement on the basis on which you will carry out your review and I am sure it will prove a most important contribution to the development of health and social policy. I am extremely grateful to you for agreeing to take this on and hope we can keep in touch from time to time in the months ahead.

TESSA JOWELL

The Process of the Inquiry

1. Sir Donald Acheson was invited by Ministers on 10 July 1997 to undertake an independent review of inequalities of health in England. The commissioning letter from the Minister for Public Health is attached at annex A.

Terms of Reference

2. The Inquiry's terms of reference were:
   (1) To moderate a Department of Health review of the latest available information on inequalities of health, using data from the Office for National Statistics, the Department of Health and elsewhere. The data review would summarise the evidence of inequalities of health and expectation of life in England and identify trends.
   (2) In the light of that evidence, to conduct – within the broad framework of the Government's overall financial strategy – an independent review to identify priority areas for future policy development, which scientific and expert evidence indicates are likely to offer opportunities for Government to develop beneficial, cost effective and affordable interventions to reduce health inequalities.
   (3) The review will report to the Secretary of State for Health. The report will be published and its conclusions, based on evidence, will contribute to the development of a new strategy for health.

3. The purpose of the Inquiry was to inform the development of the Government's public health strategy and, in particular, to contribute to the forthcoming White Paper, "Our Healthier Nation". A two stage timescale was agreed to assist this process. It provided for confidential draft advice to be presented to Ministers in advance of the publication of the final report.

Scientific Advisory Group

4. After initial consultations on the major issues of health inequalities in the summer of 1997, the business of the Inquiry was taken forward by a Scientific Advisory Group (SAG) of experts, chaired by Sir Donald and supported by a small Secretariat. The members of the Group were:

   Professor David Barker FRS, Director of the Medical Research Council's Environmental Epidemiology Unit, University of Southampton
   Dr Jacky Chambers, Director of Public Health, Birmingham Health Authority

   Professor Hilary Graham, Director of the Economic and Social Research Council's Health Variations Programme at Lancaster University
   Professor Michael Marmot, Professor of Epidemiology and Public Health, University College, London and Director of the International Centre for Health and Society.
   Dr Margaret Whitehead, Visiting Fellow at the King's Fund, London

5. The SAG met on 19 occasions between August 1997 and September 1998. It oversaw the process, received the evidence submitted and developed the recommendations and the final report.

Process

6. As a first step, the Inquiry commissioned a series of topic (or "input") papers from academics and other experts in the field. The purpose of the papers was to identify and summarise key issues and to allow the SAG to consider the state of the scientific evidence and possible areas for policy development in accordance with the Inquiry's terms of reference.

7. The Inquiry took a broad view of the causes and the impact of health inequalities on individuals and society. Accordingly, these papers explored aspects of the life course, of the economic, social and physical environments, and of the behaviours which affect individual health. Input papers on a total of 17 topics were presented to the SAG. They are listed in full in Annex D.

8. Most of the authors of the input papers consulted widely among a network of other researchers in the area. The papers were presented at SAG meetings by the author(s). Invited experts were asked to comment on the input papers as part of the SAG discussions. The main findings of the papers and results of the SAG discussions were summarised in a series of commentaries.

9. These input papers, and commentaries, together with other evidence were scrutinised by a separate Evaluation Group. This Group, chaired by Professor Sally Macintyre, Director of the MRC Medical Sociology Unit, was set up to provide a further element of peer review to the process. The members of the Group were Dr Iain Chalmers, Director of the UK Cochrane Centre, Dr Richard Horton, editor of *The Lancet*, Dr Richard Smith, editor of the *British Medical Journal*. The Group noted the lack of evidence to support many

suggested policy interventions, and recommended that the Inquiry should make explicit the quality of evidence and argument used to support proposed areas for policy development. The SAG received a report from the Group and accepted its advice.

10. The SAG also received a number of presentations from other experts and from within its own ranks. These were usually less formal events, and the results were not considered by the Evaluation Group. They were, nevertheless, crucial in expanding and strengthening the evidence base of the Inquiry.

11. Written submissions were also sought from a range of bodies and individuals, and many additional contributions were received. This evidence was considered by the SAG and, as far as possible, fed into the development and review of the input papers. A full list of the presentations and submissions received is in annex D.

12. The process was also aided by a series of "chairman's briefings", usually informal discussions with experts covering issues arising from the consultation paper "Our Healthier Nation" and from the initiatives of other Government Departments.

13. The report's recommendations and supporting argument documented in this report are the result of all these processes.

14. Draft confidential advice was submitted to Ministers in July. This final report was submitted at the end of September 1998

Acknowledgements

The Inquiry would like to thank the many individuals and organisations who provided valuable information and support across the wide range of our interests.

Iain Chalmers was a founding member of the Scientific Advisory Group (SAG) and resigned after the early meetings to concentrate on supporting the Evaluation Group. He was aided by Trevor Sheldon until he left the SAG. The SAG was also aided by David Blane and Cyrus Cooper who served as substitutes for Michael Marmot and David Barker in the early months of the Inquiry.

The secretariat to the Inquiry was provided by Ray Earwicker (Administrative Secretary) and Catherine Law (Scientific Secretary). Frances Drever was the Statistical Adviser to the Inquiry. Anna Donald and James Nazroo assisted with scientific aspects of the work. Scientific support was also provided by Malu Drachler, Kerry-Ann Holder and Tanja Megens. Zubeda Seedat provided administrative support for the team. Gabrielle Allnut, Gavin Larner and Imogen O'Shea provided Secretariat support in the early months of the Inquiry. Jane Kincaid was Sir Donald's personal secretary during the Inquiry. Jane Pearce provided secretarial support to Catherine Law.

Sally Macintyre chaired the Evaluation Group. The other members were Iain Chalmers, Richard Horton, and Richard Smith.

Input papers were commissioned by the Inquiry from experts in the field. They were Sara Arber, Michaela Benzeval, Richard Best, David Blane, George Davey Smith, Adrian Davis, Anna Donald, David Goldberg, Bobbie Jacobson, Kay-Tee Khaw, Catherine Law, Barbara MacGibbon, Sally Macintyre, James Nazroo, Michael Nelson, Aubrey Sheiham (together with Richard Watt), and, Jane Wardle (together with Michael Farrell, Mervyn Hillsdon, Martin Jarvis, Stephen Sutton and Margaret Thorogood), Patrick West, Richard Wilkinson, Geoff Whitty (together with Peter Aggleton, Eva Gamarnikow and Paul Tyrer).

The discussion of these papers within the SAG was informed by contributions from: Mel Bartley, Raj Bhopal, Liza Catan, Sarah Curtis, Astrid Fletcher, David Gordon, Bobbie Jacobson, Michael Joffe, Suzi Leather, David Leon, Stuart Logan, Duncan Maclennan, Alan Marsh, Chris Power, Andrew Rugg Gunn, Helen Sweeting, Chris Thompson, and Sally Tomlinson.

The following individuals provided valuable assistance to the Inquiry: Phil Alderson, Eric Appleby, Jim Appleyard, John Ashton, Rasaratnam Balajaran, Sir Christopher Ball, Terri Banks, Ann Barker, Colin Barnes, John Bennett, Richard Berthoud, Roger Bibbings, Sheila Bingham, Sir Douglas Black, Mildred Blaxter, Lisa Bostock, Shaun Boyle, Michael Chan, David Coggon, Michel Coleman, Sarah Colles, June Crown, Göran Dahlgren, Nick Day, Finn Diderichsen, Sir Richard Doll, Peter Flynn, Kamini Gadhok, Jane Gillie, John Gooderham, John Gray, Sian Griffiths, Sir John Grimley-Evans, David Hall, Chris Ham, Mike Hayes, Iona Heath, Kate Hunt, Raymond Illsley, Rachel Jenkins, Ken Judge, John Keast, Sebastian Kramer, Ramesh Kumar, Tim Lang, Gaynor Legall, David Lewis, David Lindsay, Robert Maxwell, Martin McKee, Pamela Meadows, Geof Mercer, Lynn Murray, Fraser Mustard, Julia Neuberger, Anne Parker, Marie Power, Andrew Prentice, George Radda, Hamid Rehman, Sian Robinson, Ian Roberts, Helen Roberts, Roberto Rona, Sir Michael Rutter, Alex Scott Samuel, Carol Sherriff, Anne Sofer, Tony Stanton, Carolyn Stephens, Sarah Stewart-Brown, Sir Kenneth Stowe, Peter Townsend, David Weaver, and John Yates.

Written submissions were sought from a range of organisations and individuals, and many additional contributions were received. A list of contributors is attached at Annex D.

Officials from several different Government Departments not listed individually provided the Inquiry with information, assistance and advice.

The Inquiry was supported by the Department of Health who provided office accommodation and support staff.

The Medical Research Council provided the Scientific Secretary and support staff from its Environmental Epidemiology Unit at the University of Southampton.

Papers, Submissions and Evidence to the Inquiry

Input Papers

The SAG received and discussed the following commissioned input papers, listed below.

1. **Mothers/families/children**
   Catherine Law, MRC Environmental Epidemiology Unit, University of Southampton

2. **Youth**
   Patrick West, MRC Medical Sociology Unit, Glasgow

3. **Adults of Working Age**
   David Blane, Imperial College, London

4. **Older People**
   Kay-Tee Khaw, University of Cambridge

5. **Housing**
   Richard Best, Joseph Rowntree Foundation

6. **Social Environment**
   Richard Wilkinson, University of Sussex

7. **Poverty and Income**
   George Davey Smith, University of Bristol

8. **National Health Service**
   (a) Michaela Benzeval, King's Fund and Anna Donald, University College, London
   (b) Bobbie Jacobson, City and East London Health Authority

9. **Nutrition**
   Michael Nelson, King's College, London

10. **Education**
    Geoff Whitty, Institute of Education, London (lead author)

11. **Areas**
    Sally Macintyre, MRC Medical Sociology Unit, Glasgow

12. **Ethnicity**
    James Nazroo, Policy Studies Institute, London

13. **Transport/Pollution/Material Environment**
    (a) Adrian Davies, Open University
    (b) Barbara MacGibbon, MRC Institute for Environment and Health, Leicester

14. **Gender**
    Sara Arber, University of Surrey

15. **Mental Health**
    Sir David Goldberg, Institute of Psychiatry, London

16. **Health-Related Behaviours**
    Jane Wardle, University College, London (lead author)

17. **Oral Health**
    Aubrey Sheiham, University College, London (lead author)

Other Presentations

The SAG received a number of other presentations and briefings from experts in the field, apart from those provided by Departmental officials. They were:

Policies to Tackle Inequalities in Health, Margaret Whitehead, King's Fund

Socioeconomic Determinants and Ill Health, Andrew Dilnot, Institute for Fiscal Studies and Richard Wilkinson, University of Sussex

Area Inequalities, Daniel Dorling, University of Bristol, and John Hills, Centre for Analysis of Social Exclusion, London School of Economics

Life Cycle Trajectories, Diana Kuh, Chris Power, Yoav Ben-Shlomo and Mike Wadsworth, University College, London

Socioeconomic Discussion Paper, Hilary Graham, ESRC Health Variations Programme, Lancaster University, Michael Marmot, University College, London

The Role of Pyschosocial Factors, The MacArthur Foundation Research Network on Socioeconomic Status and Health, Teresa Seeman, Sheldon Cohen, Shelley Taylor, Karen Mathews, and Michael Marmot

Psychosocial Stress in Childhood, Scott Montgomery, Royal Free Hospital School of Medicine, London

Intergenerational Effects on Inequalities in Health, David Barker, MRC Environmental Epidemiology Unit, University of Southampton

Stress in the Workplace, Peter Graham and Malcolm Darvill, Health Directorate, Health and Safety Executive and David Coggon, MRC Environmental Epidemiology Unit, University of Southampton

Benefits Briefing, John Hills, Centre for Analysis of Social Exclusion, London School of Economics, and Robert Walker, Centre for Social Policy Research, Loughborough University

Health Inequalities at a Local Level, Jacky Chambers, Birmingham Health Authority, Ruth Hussey, Director of Public Health, Liverpool Health Authority, Alan Chape, Deputy Chief Executive, Liverpool City Council, Bob Stewart, Newcastle Healthy Cities

Submissions

The following individuals submitted evidence to the Inquiry:

Jo Asvall, Christopher Bates, Peter Bradley, Eric Brunner, Mike Catchpole, Ben Cave, Elizabeth Dowler, Douglas Fleming, Peter Fonagy, John Godfrey, Meg Goodman, Mark Haggard, Andrew Haines, Irene Higginson, Anthony Jenner, Colwyn Jones, Brian Keeble, Azim Lakhani, Alyson Learmonth, Gerard Leavey, Michael Lennon, Donald Light, Caroline Lindsey, Paul Nicholson, John Radford, Bethan Reeves, Jane Robinson, Michael Rosen, Oliver Russell, John Shanks, Veena Soni Raleigh, Marjorie Smith, Simon Strickland, Kathy Sylva, Jonathan Talbot, Mary Tilki, Patricia Walls, Graham Watt, Elizabeth Whitehead, Arthur Wynn, Margaret Wynn.

The following organisations submitted evidence to the Inquiry

Action on Smoking and Health (ASH), ASH Scotland, and ASH Wales
Afiya Trust
Age Concern
Alcohol Concern
Association for Public Health
Association of Charity Officers
Association of Community Health Councils
Association of Directors of Social Services
Barnados
British Medical Association
Centre for Health Economics, University of York
Chartered Institute of Environmental Health
Child Accident Prevention Trust
Child Health Advocacy Network and the National Children's Bureau
Child Psychotherapy Trust
Community Practitioners' and Health Visitors' Association
Coventry City Council
Derby City Council
Economic and Social Research Council
EQUAL
Equal Opportunities Commission
Faculty of Public Health Medicine
Faculty of Occupational Medicine and Society of Occupational Medicine
Family Planning Association
Food and Drink Federation
Friends of the Earth
Health and Low Income Project
Health Education Authority
Institute of Child Health
Inter-Authority Comparisons and Consultancy
King's Fund
Kirklees Health for All Women Health Policy Group
Kirklees Metropolitan Authority
Local Government Association
London School of Hygiene and Tropical Medicine
Macmillan Cancer Relief

Medical Practitioners' Union
Medical Research Council
Men's Health Forum
Men's Health Trust
MIND
National Energy Action
National Food Alliance
National Heart Forum
National Institute for Ethnic Studies in Health and Social Policy
National Institute for Social Work
National Osteoporosis Society
National Perinatal Epidemiology Unit
NHS Confederation
North West Public Health Association
Nutrition Society
Oxfam
Peak District Rural Deprivation Forum
Public Health Alliance
Public Health Laboratory Service
Royal of Pathologists
Royal College of Opthalmologists
Royal College of Physicians
Royal College of Psychiatrists
Royal College of Surgeons
Royal College of Midwives
Royal College of Nursing
Royal College of Paediatrics and Child Health
Royal College of Obstetricians and Gynaecologists
Royal College of General Practitioners
Sheffield City Council
Sheffield Health
Shelter
Socialist Health Association
Society of Health Promotion Specialists Poverty Caucus Group
Society for Social Medicine
Stroke Association
The Big Issue in the North and the Big Step Limited
Tobacco Control Alliance
UK Baby Friendly Initiative
Watson Wyatt Partners
West Kent Breastfeeding Alliance

INDEPENDENT INQUIRY INTO INEQUALITIES IN HEALTH

Index

Indexed by Lisa Footitt and George Curzon,
INDEXING SPECIALISTS